MCQs in Anatomy for Undergr
and Medical Students

MCQs in Anatomy for Undergraduates and Medical Students

M. Jamil MB ChB FRCS

Specialist Registrar in Neurosurgery,
The National Hospital for Neurology and Neurosurgery,
Queen Square, London

B. S. Mitchell BSc PhD FIBMS CBiol MIBiol

Senior Lecturer in Anatomy,
Anglo-European College of Chiropractic, Bournemouth
Formerly of the Department of Human Morphology,
University of Southampton

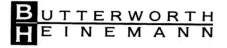

Butterworth-Heinemann Ltd
Linacre House, Jordan Hill, Oxford OX2 8DP
A division of Reed Educational and Professional Publishing Ltd

 A member of the Reed Elsevier plc group

OXFORD   BOSTON   JOHANNESBURG
MELBOURNE   NEW DELHI   SINGAPORE

First published 1997

British Library Cataloguing in Publication Data
A catalogue record for this book is available from the British Library

ISBN 0 7506 3591 6

Typeset by BC Typesetting, Bristol BS18 1NZ
Printed and bound in Great Britain by Biddles Ltd, Guildford and King's Lynn

Contents

Introduction

Anatomy underpins many biomedical disciplines and forms the basis of many professional approaches to patient care. In this book we have attempted to provide a range of questions that will help students to determine their knowledge and understanding of this important subject.

The book is deliberately aimed at a multiprofessional readership, including those studying undergraduate anatomy such as medical students, and others studying related sciences, physiotherapy, occupational therapy, osteopathy and chiropractic.

We recommend that you use this book as an adjunct to your studies. The secret of success in anatomy is to be familiar with the subject. We hope this book will help you to do so, though it is not a substitute for the numerous good textbooks that are already available.

MJ
BSM
London and
Bournemouth
January 1997

Upper limb

1. **Latissimus dorsi muscle:**
   a. Is innervated by a branch of the posterior cord of the brachial plexus.
   b. Extends the shoulder joint.
   c. Inserts into the bicipital groove of the humerus above teres minor.
   d. Prevents winging of the scapula.
   e. Arises from the spinous processes of the lower three cervical and upper six thoracic vertebrae.

2. **The rotator cuff muscles:**
   a. Are latissimus dorsi, infraspinatus, supraspinatus and subscapularis.
   b. Subscapularis is supplied by the suprascapular nerve which arises from the upper trunk of the brachial plexus.
   c. Are all powerful adductors of the shoulder joint.
   d. Attach near the shoulder joint and partly fuse with the lateral part of its capsule.

Upper limb

1. a. True It is supplied by the thoracodorsal nerve (nerve to latissimus dorsi) which arises from the posterior cord.
   b. True It is also a powerful adductor and medial rotator of the shoulder joint.
   c. False It does insert into the bicipital groove. However, it is inserted between pectoralis major and teres major. A useful *aide-mémoire*: Lady Di is protected by two majors – latissimus dorsi (Lady Di), pectoralis major and teres major.
   d. False It is serratus anterior that prevents winging of the scapula, which could occur if there is damage to the long thoracic nerve due to action of the other scapular muscles.
   e. False It arises from the spinous processes, and supraspinous ligaments of the lower six thoracic vertebrae, and all the lumbar and sacral vertebrae. It also arises from the iliac crest, and the lowest four ribs.

2. a. False They are teres minor, infraspinatus, supraspinatus and subscapularis, and can be remembered by their acronym TISS.
   b. False It is supraspinatus and infraspinatus which are supplied by the suprascapular nerve; subscapularis is supplied by the upper and lower subscapular nerves which arise from the posterior cord.
   c. False Teres minor is a weak adductor of the shoulder. Supraspinatus is an abductor of the shoulder joint, infraspinatus is a lateral rotator and subscapularis is a medial rotator of the humerus. They all act together to brace the head of the humerus against the glenoid fossa, and provide stability of the joint in movements of the distal parts of the upper limb.
   d. True It is by this mechanism that they provide support and stability to the shoulder joint.

3. **In the upper limb:**
   a. The ulnar nerve lies under flexor carpi ulnaris on flexor digitorum superficialis.
   b. The median nerve gives a branch to the thenar muscles which runs superficial to the flexor retinaculum.
   c. The ulnar nerve usually supplies flexor carpi ulnaris and the ulnar half of flexor digitorum superficialis.
   d. The median nerve passes between the two heads of pronator teres and passes distally under flexor digitorum superficialis.
   e. The radial artery gives off the posterior interosseous artery which supplies the extensor compartment of the forearm.

4. **In movement at the shoulder joint:**
   a. Adduction is achieved mainly by pectoralis major, latissimus dorsi and deltoid.
   b. Abduction is initiated by supraspinatus which acts with the acromial fibres of deltoid.
   c. Pectoralis minor plays an important role in flexion.
   d. The lateral and medial heads of triceps extend the joint.
   e. All the rotators of the shoulder are supplied by branches of the brachial plexus.

3. a. False It lies between flexor carpi ulnaris and flexor digitorum profundus.
  b. False It is the branch from the median nerve supplying the skin over the thenar muscles which passes superficial to the flexor retinaculum. The branch supplying the muscles passes deep to it. This explains the wasting of the thenar eminence seen in carpal tunnel syndrome.
  c. False It supplies flexor carpi ulnaris and the ulnar half of flexor digitorum profundus. Flexor digitorum superficialis is supplied by the median nerve.
  d. True It also supplies both these muscles.
  e. False Both the anterior and posterior interosseous arteries arise from the common interosseous artery which is a branch of the ulnar artery.

4. a. False Deltoid is an abductor of the shoulder joint.
  b. True The teres muscles are also involved. They pull down the head of the humerus to counteract the upwards pull of the contracting fibres of deltoid.
  c. False It plays a role in protraction of the scapula through its insertion on the coracoid process.
  d. False They are extensors of the elbow. The **long** head aids in extending the shoulder.
  e. True No muscle acting on the shoulder joint is supplied by any nerve above C_5 or below T_1 which is the root value of the brachial plexus.

5. At the wrist:
   a. The triquetral bone lies in the distal row of carpal bones on the radial side of the lunate.
   b. The trapezoid articulates with the thumb metacarpal.
   c. Ossification of the capitate is a sign that the fetus is full-term (gestational age over 38 weeks).
   d. The styloid process of the radius is distal to the styloid process of the ulna.
   e. The proximal and distal palmar creases overlie the flexor retinaculum.

6. Pectoralis major:
   a. With latissimus dorsi, forms the anterior axillary fold.
   b. Has a clavicular head which arises from the middle third of the clavicle.
   c. Has costal elements which arise from the upper six costal cartilages.
   d. Is supplied by all five segments of the brachial plexus.
   e. Can be an accessory muscle of respiration.

7. Pectoralis minor:
   a. Arises from the third, fourth and fifth costal cartilages.
   b. Is inserted into the acromion process.
   c. Is supplied by both pectoral nerves which arise from the posterior cord of the brachial plexus.
   d. Overlies the axillary artery, which it divides into three parts.
   e. Overlies the roots of the brachial plexus.

5. a. False The triquetral bone lies in the distal row of carpal bones on the ulnar aspect of the lunate. A good mnemonic for the carpal bones is: sexy Lucy tried parking, having crashed twenty times – scaphoid, lunate, triquetral, pisiform, hamate, capitate, trapezoid, trapezium. Once again, the original mnemonic has been amended slightly in the interests of good taste. The sequence of the bones in this case starts on the radial aspect and goes round in a circular fashion.

b. False It is the trapezium which articulates with the thumb metacarpal. The mnemonic above does not differentiate between the two Ts – trapezoid and trapezium. A useful little rhyme is: the trapezium lies under the thumb.

c. False None of the carpal bones has ossified at birth.

d. True The radial styloid can extend almost 2 cm beyond the ulnar styloid.

e. False The flexor retinaculum lies much further distally. The distal palmar crease overlies the proximal border of the flexor retinaculum.

6. a. False Latissimus dorsi lies in the posterior axillary fold.

b. False The clavicular head arises from the medial half of the clavicle.

c. True Pectoralis major also has fibres which arise from the sternum.

d. True $C_{5,6}$ supply the clavicular head, and $C_{7,8}T_1$ supply the sternocostal part.

e. True It is attached to the chest wall and the humerus. If one is fixed, the other must move.

7. a. False It arises from the third, fourth and fifth *ribs*.

b. False It is inserted into the coracoid process.

c. False It is supplied by both pectoral nerves. The medial pectoral nerve arises from the medial cord of the brachial plexus and the lateral pectoral nerve arises from the lateral cord.

d. True The first part of the axillary artery lies above pectoralis minor, the second part lies behind it, and the third part lies inferior to it.

e. False It overlies the *cords* of the brachial plexus.

8. **The axillary artery:**
   a. Is the direct continuation of the third part of the subclavian artery.
   b. Becomes the brachial artery when it emerges inferior to pectoralis minor.
   c. Has the three cords of the brachial plexus embracing its second part.
   d. Has no branches from its first part.
   e. Has the internal thoracic artery arising from its second part.

9. **Trapezius:**
   a. Is supplied from the posterior cord of the brachial plexus.
   b. Has fibres which take origin from the skull.
   c. Inserts entirely on to the scapula.
   d. Is assisted in its action by serratus anterior and levator scapulae.
   e. Takes origin from the spinous processes and supraspinous ligaments of the upper six thoracic vertebrae.

10. **Serratus anterior:**
    a. Arises by four digitations arising from the upper four ribs.
    b. Has all its digitations inserting into the scapula.
    c. Is supplied by the long thoracic nerve (nerve to serratus anterior) which has a root value of $C_{7,8}T_1$.
    d. Has its nerve supply arising directly from the roots of the brachial plexus.
    e. Is tested by asking the patient to push against a wall.

8. a. True   The subclavian artery becomes the axillary artery at the outer border of the first rib.

   b. False   It becomes the brachial artery at the lower border of teres major.

   c. True   The three cords of the brachial plexus embrace the second part of the axillary artery and are named medial, lateral and posterior according to their position in relation to it.

   d. False   The superior thoracic artery which supplies both pectoral muscles arises from the first part of the axillary artery.

   e. False   The internal thoracic artery arises from the first part of the subclavian artery.

9. a. False   It is supplied by the accessory (11th cranial) nerve.

   b. True   It has fibres which arise from the superior nuchal line on the occipital bone.

   c. False   It has fibres which insert into the lateral part of the clavicle.

   d. True   These two muscles also elevate, rotate and stabilize the scapula.

   e. False   It takes origin from the spinous processes and supraspinous ligaments of all 12 thoracic vertebrae.

10. a. False   It has eight digitations which arise from the upper eight ribs, interdigitating with the origin of the external oblique muscle.

   b. True   The first two insert into the upper angle of the scapula, the third and fourth into the deep surface of the medial border of the scapula, and the lower four digitations into the inferior angle of the scapula.

   c. False   The long thoracic nerve arises from the C_{5-7} roots.

   d. True   The other two nerves which arise directly from the roots of the brachial plexus are the dorsal scapular nerve (nerve to the rhomboids) and the nerve to subclavius.

   e. True   Paralysis will give rise to the classical sign of winging of the scapula.

11. The sternoclavicular joint:
  a.   Is an atypical synovial joint.
  b.   Is strengthened by the interclavicular ligament which joins the upper part of the sternal ends of the two clavicles together and is attached to the body of the sternum at the jugular notch.
  c.   Is supplied by the medial supraclavicular nerves from the cervical plexus.
  d.   Is strengthened by anterior and posterior sternoclavicular ligaments which are the major stabilizing factor preventing dislocation of the joint.

12. The acromioclavicular joint:
  a.   Is a fibrous joint between the lateral end of the clavicle and the medial end of the acromion process of the scapula.
  b.   Is strengthened by the acromioclavicular ligament, which is the main factor in its stability.
  c.   Is also stabilized by the coracoclavicular ligament which consists of two parts – conoid and trapezoid.
  d.   Is also supplied from the cervical plexus.

13. The axilla:
  a.   Has a floor which is supported by the suspensory ligament which arises from the lower border of subclavius.
  b.   Has a posterior wall made up of the tendon of latissimus dorsi and the medial head of triceps.
  c.   Has a lateral wall formed by the shaft of the humerus.
  d.   Contains the roots of the brachial plexus.
  e.   Has the axillary vein which lies between the artery and the brachial plexus.

11. a. True It is atypical because it contains a fibrocartilaginous disc.
   b. False The interclavicular ligament is attached to the *manubrium sterni* at the jugular notch.
   c. True Their root value is C_3 and C_4.
   d. False The major stabilizing factor preventing dislocation is the costoclavicular ligament. The anterior and posterior sternoclavicular ligaments are merely thickenings in the capsule of the joint.

12. a. False It is another atypical synovial joint.
   b. False It is the coracoclavicular ligament which is the main provider of stability to the acromioclavicular joint.
   c. True The conoid ligament is attached to the conoid tubercle on the clavicle, and the trapezoid ligament attaches to the inferior surface of the lateral aspect of the clavicle. Both arise from the coracoid process.
   d. True It receives its nerve supply from the lateral supraclavicular nerves which arise from the C_4 nerve root.

13. a. False The suspensory ligament is attached to the lower border of *pectoralis minor*.
   b. False The posterior wall of the axilla is made up of subscapularis, teres major and the tendon of latissimus dorsi.
   c. True The anterior fold (mainly pectoralis major) and the posterior fold (mainly latissimus dorsi) converge on the humerus and are both inserted on to its medial surface, thus delineating the lateral wall of the axilla.
   d. False It is the *cords* of the brachial plexus which are present in the axilla.
   e. False The cords of the brachial plexus embrace the axillary artery. The axillary vein lies medial to them both.

14. Subscapularis:
    a. Arises from the inner surface of the scapula.
    b. Inserts into the greater tuberosity of the humerus.
    c. Holds the scapula down against the chest wall.
    d. Is supplied from the posterior cord of the brachial plexus.
    e. Is a lateral rotator of the shoulder joint.

15. Teres major:
    a. Arises from the inner surface of the lateral border of the scapula.
    b. Lies above teres minor.
    c. Inserts into the medial aspect of the humerus.
    d. Is supplied by the dorsal scapular nerve.
    e. Plays a role in stabilizing the shoulder joint.

16. The muscular spaces in the arm include:
    a. The quadrilateral space (quadrangular space), which transmits the radial nerve.
    b. The triangular space, which is bounded by the long head of triceps medially, the shaft of the humerus laterally and subscapularis above.
    c. The quadrilateral space, which transmits the posterior circumflex humeral artery.
    d. A second triangular space, which lies medial to the quadrilateral space and transmits no nerve.
    e. The quadrilateral space, which has subscapularis as its upper border if viewed from the inside, and teres major as its upper border if viewed from behind.

14. a. True   This is obvious from its name.
   b. False   It inserts into the lesser tuberosity of the humerus and the area just below it.
   c. False   Subscapularis cannot perform this action as it has no attachment to the chest wall. Serratus anterior holds the scapula to the chest wall.
   d. True   This is via the upper and lower subscapular nerves.
   e. False   It is a *medial* rotator of the shoulder joint. It is part of the rotator cuff group of muscles, comprising subscapularis, supraspinatus, infraspinatus and teres minor, which stabilize the shoulder joint.

15. a. False   It arises from the *dorsal* surface of the lateral border of the scapula. The inner surface provides origin for the fibres of subscapularis.
   b. False   The muscle which lies above teres minor is infraspinatus. Teres major lies inferior to it.
   c. True   It is obvious therefore that it will adduct the abducted arm.
   d. False   The dorsal scapular nerve is the nerve to the rhomboids. Teres major is supplied by the lower subscapular nerve.
   e. True   Even though it is not one of the four rotator cuff muscles (see Upper limb question 2), its insertion into the upper humerus helps in steadying the head of the humerus and keeping it within the glenoid fossa.

16. a. False   It is the axillary nerve which passes through the quadrangular space accompanied by the posterior circumflex humeral artery. The radial nerve passes through the triangular space along with the profunda brachii artery.
   b. False   The borders of the triangular space are the long head of triceps medially, the shaft of the humerus laterally and teres major above.
   c. True   It accompanies the axillary nerve.
   d. True   This space has less clinical significance as it only transmits the circumflex scapular artery.
   e. False   When viewed from behind, teres *minor* forms the upper border of the quadrilateral space. Teres major always forms its lower border.

Upper limb

17. The axillary artery:
   a. Enters the axilla by passing between pectoralis major and pectoralis minor.
   b. Has the two heads of the median nerve embracing its first part.
   c. Has three branches arising from its first part, all of which supply the anterior chest wall.
   d. Gives off the anterior circumflex humeral artery which passes through the quadrilateral space with the radial nerve.
   e. Has three branches arising from its third part: the anterior and posterior circumflex humeral arteries, and the circumflex scapular artery.

18. The axillary vein:
   a. Is firmly enclosed in the axillary sheath.
   b. Is formed by the union of the venae comitantes accompanying the brachial artery.
   c. Passes in front of scalenus anterior.
   d. Grooves the inferior surface of the first rib.
   e. Is an ideal site for insertion of a central venous line.

14

17. a. False The axillary artery lies deep to both pectoral
muscles. It passes underneath pectoralis minor
which divides it into its three parts.

b. False The cords of the brachial plexus embrace the
second part of the axillary artery, and the two
heads of the median nerve embrace its *third* part.

c. False The first part of the axillary artery has only one
branch – the superior thoracic artery which supplies
both pectoral muscles.

d. False It is the *posterior* circumflex humeral artery which
passes through the quadrilateral space. It is
accompanied by the axillary nerve. The radial nerve
passes through the triangular space.

e. False The branches of the third part of the axillary artery
are the anterior and posterior circumflex humeral
arteries and the subscapular artery. The circumflex
scapular artery is a branch of the subscapular
artery.

18. a. False The vein lies outside the sheath, thus allowing for
distension with increased venous return. This occurs
during periods of increased muscular activity in the
upper limb.

b. True The basilic and cephalic veins drain into it.

c. False Scalenus anterior inserts into the first rib. At the
outer border of the first rib, the axillary vein has
by definition become the subclavian vein. It is
therefore the subclavian vein which lies in front of
scalenus anterior.

d. False There is a groove on the *superior* surface of the first
rib. It is debatable whether this groove is caused by
the subclavian artery, vein or lower trunk of the
brachial plexus.

e. False The axilla is certainly not the most comfortable,
nor the cleanest of sites for a central venous line.
The subclavian or internal jugular veins are the
ones usually cannulated when central venous access
is required.

19. Biceps brachii:
   a. Arises via two heads which usually fuse proximal to the elbow joint.
   b. Is inserted mainly into the interosseous membrane which joins the radius and ulna.
   c. Is the main flexor of the elbow.
   d. Assists pronator teres and pronator quadratus in pronating the forearm.
   e. Has the median nerve supplying its long head and the ulnar nerve supplying its short head.

20. The brachial plexus:
   a. Supplies the erector spinae muscles segmentally via its posterior roots.
   b. Supplies the flexors of the upper limbs from its anterior divisions.
   c. Has its three cords lying behind scalenus anterior.
   d. Has three branches arising from its anterior and posterior divisions.
   e. Has a medial cord which receives a contribution from each of the five nerve roots which make up the brachial plexus.

19. a. True The two heads are sometimes found fused high up in the arm.
 b. False It is inserted into the radial tuberosity via its distal tendon, and into the deep fascia of the forearm via its bicipital aponeurosis.
 c. True As it contracts, it pulls on the tuberosity of the radius, thus flexing the elbow.
 d. False It is obvious from its insertion that it is a supinator of the forearm, but only when the elbow is flexed.
 e. False This is total rubbish! Both heads of biceps brachii are supplied by the musculocutaneous nerve.

20. a. False The brachial plexus is formed by the anterior rami of C_5–T_1. The erector spinae muscles are innervated segmentally by the posterior rami of the spinal nerves.
 b. True The flexors are supplied by the anterior divisions and the extensors are supplied by the posterior divisions.
 c. False The trunks of the brachial plexus lie behind scalenus anterior. The cords lie in the axilla.
 d. False There are no branches arising from the divisions.
 e. False The medial cord is the continuation of the anterior division of the lower trunk which arises from C_8 and T_1 nerve roots only.

21. The branches of the brachial plexus include:
  a. Three supraclavicular branches, which are the upper and lower subscapular nerves and the nerve to subclavius.
  b. The suprascapular nerve, which is the only branch from the divisions.
  c. The musculocutaneous nerve, which arises from the lateral cord and supplies coracobrachialis.
  d. The ulnar nerve, which is the largest branch of the posterior cord.
  e. The thoracodorsal nerve, which arises from the upper trunk.

22. In the shoulder region:
  a. There are six muscles arising from the scapula which are inserted into the humerus.
  b. Supraspinatus, infraspinatus and teres minor arise from the dorsal surface of the scapula and are inserted into the lesser tuberosity of the humerus.
  c. Trapezius overlies the rotator cuff and inserts distally on to the lateral aspect of the shaft of the humerus.
  d. Abduction is initiated by trapezius and completed by deltoid.
  e. The joint is supplied by twigs from the median, ulnar and radial nerves.

21. a. False The supraclavicular branches are the branches from the roots. They are the dorsal scapular nerve (nerve to the rhomboids), the nerve to subclavius and the long thoracic nerve (nerve to serratus anterior). Be careful not to confuse the supraclavicular branches of the brachial plexus with the supraclavicular nerves which are derived from the cervical plexus.

b. False There are no branches from the divisions. The suprascapular nerve is the only branch from the *trunks*.

c. True It also supplies biceps brachii and brachialis and is sensory to the lateral aspect of the forearm via the lateral cutaneous nerve of the forearm.

d. False The ulnar nerve arises from the *medial* cord. It is the radial nerve which is the largest branch of the posterior cord.

e. False The thoracodorsal nerve (nerve to latissimus dorsi) arises from the posterior cord. It is the *suprascapular* nerve which arises from the upper trunk.

22. a. True They are supraspinatus, infraspinatus, teres major, teres minor, subscapularis and deltoid. With the exception of teres major and deltoid, these muscles form the rotator cuff which stabilizes the shoulder joint.

b. False They all insert into the *greater* tuberosity of the humerus.

c. False Trapezius inserts into the spine of the scapula and has no attachment on the humerus.

d. False Abduction is initiated by *supraspinatus* and completed by deltoid.

e. False These nerves do *not* supply the muscles which move the shoulder. According to Hilton's law, the shoulder is supplied by the axillary, musculocutaneous and suprascapular nerves.

23. Supraspinatus:
  a.   Is one of the rotator cuff muscles.
  b.   Has a tendon which blends with the capsule of the shoulder joint.
  c.   Is supplied by the dorsal scapular nerve which arises from the posterior cord of the brachial plexus.
  d.   Plays a role in preventing dislocation of the shoulder joint.
  e.   Is an adductor of the shoulder joint.

24. Infraspinatus:
  a.   Arises from the ventral surface of the scapula.
  b.   Gives rise to a tendon which blends with the capsule of the shoulder joint, thus strengthening it.
  c.   Is supplied by the suprascapular nerve.
  d.   Is a medial rotator of the shoulder joint.
  e.   Lies deep to trapezius.

25. Teres minor:
  a.   Arises from the lateral margin of the dorsal aspect of the scapula.
  b.   Inserts into the lower part of the greater tuberosity of the humerus.
  c.   Is supplied by the suprascapular nerve.
  d.   Is a lateral rotator and weak adductor of the shoulder joint.
  e.   Forms the lower border of the quadrilateral space when viewed from behind.

23. a. True The others are infraspinatus, teres minor and
              subscapularis (TISS).
    b. True This strengthens the capsule of the shoulder joint.
    c. False It is supplied by the suprascapular nerve, which is
              the only branch arising from the trunks of the
              brachial plexus. It arises from the upper trunk.
    d. True This is a role it has in common with all the muscles
              of the rotator cuff.
    e. False Since the muscle arises from the supraspinous fossa
              and is inserted into the greater tuberosity of the
              humerus, it is obvious that its contraction will
              abduct the arm.

24. a. False It is *subscapularis* which arises from the ventral
              surface of the scapula. Infraspinatus arises from the
              infraspinous fossa on the *dorsal* surface of the
              latter.
    b. True This is similar to the blending which occurs
              between the tendon of supraspinatus and the
              capsule of the shoulder joint.
    c. True The suprascapular nerve supplies both
              supraspinatus and infraspinatus.
    d. False As it arises from below the spine of the scapula
              and inserts into the greater tuberosity of the
              humerus, it is obvious that its contraction would
              rotate the humerus *laterally*.
    e. True Trapezius is superficial and overlies the scapular
              muscles.

25. a. True It arises above teres major and runs parallel to the
              lower border of infraspinatus.
    b. True Supraspinatus and infraspinatus insert above it.
    c. False The suprascapular nerve supplies supraspinatus and
              infraspinatus. Teres minor is supplied by a branch
              of the axillary nerve.
    d. True It also stabilizes the shoulder joint.
    e. False When viewed from behind, teres minor forms the
              upper border of the quadrilateral space. Teres
              major forms the lower border. When viewed from
              the front, subscapularis replaces teres minor in
              forming the upper border.

26. The deltoid:
  a. Arises from a U-shaped origin on the lateral part of the clavicle, the acromion process and the lateral part of the spine of the scapula.
  b. Inserts into the lateral aspect of the shaft of the humerus.
  c. Is supplied by the axillary nerve which has a root value of $C_{7,8}$.
  d. Has anterior fibres which flex the shoulder and posterior fibres which extend it.
  e. Is the main adductor of the shoulder joint.

27. The shoulder joint:
  a. Is a synovial joint between the head of the humerus and the glenoid fossa of the scapula, which is significantly larger and holds the head of the humerus firmly within its cavity, thus preventing dislocation of the shoulder.
  b. Has a thick capsule which forms the ligament joining the two tuberosities of the humerus.
  c. Has the tendon of the short head of biceps brachii within its synovial cavity.
  d. Can only be abducted fully after medial rotation of the humerus.
  e. Is supported from above by the coracoacromial arch which fractures easily in a fall on an outstretched hand.

26. a. True Its fibres cover the shoulder joint completely.
    b. True Its fibres insert into the deltoid tuberosity of the humerus.
    c. False It is supplied by the axillary nerve, but its root value is $C_{5,6}$.
    d. True The anterior fibres arise from the clavicle and insert into the deltoid tuberosity of the humerus. They obviously flex the shoulder. The posterior fibres arise from the spine of the scapula and insert into the deltoid tuberosity, and they would obviously extend the shoulder.
    e. False It is the main *abductor* of the shoulder.

27. a. False The head of the humerus has a much larger articular surface and therefore easily slips out of the glenoid cavity.
    b. True This is the transverse ligament which joins the greater and lesser tuberosities of the humerus. It converts the bicipital groove into a canal which contains the tendon of the long head of biceps brachii.
    c. False It is the tendon of the *long* head of biceps brachii which lies within the shoulder joint.
    d. False Abduct your arm to 90°, rotate it medially, and you will note that you are unable to abduct it any further. If however you rotate it *laterally*, you will be able to abduct it further and thus raise it above your head.
    e. False The coracoacromial arch is very strong, and rarely fractured. A fall on to an outstretched hand is more likely to fracture the clavicle or the humerus or dislocate the shoulder.

28. Coracobrachialis:
   a. Arises from the coracoid process and inserts into the medial aspect of the shaft of the humerus.
   b. Adducts the shoulder.
   c. Is supplied by both medial and lateral pectoral nerves.
   d. Assists pectoralis major in raising the arm above the head.
   e. Is often found completely fused with pectoralis minor.

29. Brachialis:
   a. Arises from the inferior margin of the glenoid cavity.
   b. Is inserted into the lateral aspect of the upper one-third of the radius.
   c. Is principally a supinator of the forearm.
   d. Is supplied mainly by the musculocutaneous nerve.

30. The brachial artery:
   a. Lies medial to the median nerve at the level of the elbow.
   b. Gives off the circumflex scapular artery which supplies the infraspinous fossa.
   c. Gives off the anterior and posterior circumflex humeral arteries which accompany the axillary nerve through the quadrilateral space.
   d. Is usually accompanied by two or more venae comitantes which join to form the axillary vein.
   e. Gives off the profunda brachii artery which accompanies the ulnar nerve through the triangular space.

28. a. True It shares its origin with the short head of biceps brachii.
   b. True It is a weak adductor of the shoulder.
   c. False It is supplied by the musculocutaneous nerve which pierces it.
   d. False Raising the arm above the head involves either abduction and lateral rotation, or flexion. Coracobrachialis is not involved in any of these movements.
   e. False Although pectoralis minor is also attached to the coracoid process, it arises from the anterior chest wall, and the two muscles therefore lie at an angle to each other.

29. a. False It arises from the shaft of the humerus.
   b. False It inserts mainly into the upper part of the *ulna*.
   c. False It is principally a flexor of the forearm.
   d. True It can also receive a few twigs from the radial nerve.

30. a. False Of the two, the median nerve is the most medial structure at the level of the elbow joint.
   b. False The circumflex scapular artery does supply the infraspinous fossa; however, it arises from the subscapular artery which is a branch of the third part of the axillary artery.
   c. False The anterior and posterior circumflex humeral arteries do pass through the quadrilateral space with the axillary nerve. However, they arise from the third part of the axillary artery.
   d. True They are usually also joined by the basilic vein.
   e. False The profunda brachii artery accompanies the *radial* nerve through the triangular space.

31. **The musculocutaneous nerve:**
    a. Is the nerve of the flexor compartment of the arm.
    b. Supplies coracobrachialis and pectoralis minor.
    c. Arises from the lateral cord of the brachial plexus.
    d. Has a root value of $C_{7,8}$.
    e. Supplies biceps, brachialis and brachioradialis.

32. **Triceps:**
    a. Has a long head which arises from the infraglenoid tubercle of the scapula.
    b. Has a short head which arises from the coracoid process.
    c. Has two heads which arise from the shaft of the humerus.
    d. Is inserted mainly into the dorsal aspect of the head of the radius and is thus able to extend the elbow.
    e. Is paralysed when the radial nerve is damaged in fractures of the shaft of the humerus involving the spiral groove.

33. **The radial nerve:**
    a. Supplies anconeus.
    b. Has no cutaneous branches in the arm.
    c. Arises from the posterior cord of the brachial plexus and has a root value of C_5–T_1.
    d. Can be located at the elbow lying under cover of brachioradialis.
    e. Passes just behind the medial epicondyle of the ulna where it is easily palpable.

31. a. True It supplies the flexor muscles of the arm: coracobrachialis, biceps brachii and brachialis.
b. False Coracobrachialis *is* supplied by the musculocutaneous nerve; however, pectoralis minor is supplied by the medial and lateral pectoral nerves.
c. True The other branches of the lateral cord are the lateral pectoral nerve and the lateral head of the median nerve.
d. False The root value of the musculocutaneous nerve is $C_{5,6}$.
e. False The hint is in its name. Brachioradialis is supplied by the radial nerve. The other two are supplied by the musculocutaneous nerve.

32. a. True It enables triceps to extend the shoulder.
b. False It is the short head of *biceps* which arises from the coracoid process. The three heads of triceps are long, medial and lateral.
c. True These are the medial and lateral heads.
d. False It inserts into the olecranon process of the ulna.
e. False The triceps is supplied by branches of the radial nerve which are given off before it enters the spiral groove.

33. a. True It also supplies triceps and brachioradialis.
b. False It gives off the posterior cutaneous nerve of the arm which is sensory to the extensor surface of the arm.
c. True It is the largest nerve arising from the brachial plexus.
d. True This is the means of locating it during surgical operations.
e. False It is the *ulnar* nerve which passes behind the medial epicondyle of the ulna.

34. The elbow joint:
   a. Receives a small twig from the ulnar nerve as it passes behind the medial epicondyle.
   b. Is a synovial joint of the hinge type between the lower end of the humerus and the upper end of the ulna, with the head of the radius lying outside the joint cavity.
   c. Communicates with the proximal radioulnar joint.
   d. Has the annular ligament which is attached firmly to the head of the radius.
   e. Has the ulnar collateral ligament providing stability on the medial aspect of the joint.

35. The flexor compartment of the forearm:
   a. Consists of a superficial and deep layer of muscles.
   b. Has three muscles in the deep layer and they all arise from the common flexor origin.
   c. Has pronator teres, pronator quadratus and palmaris longus making up the deep layer.
   d. Has all the muscles of the superficial compartment supplied by the median nerve.
   e. Has flexor carpi radialis as the first muscle lying on the radial aspect in the superficial group.

36. Pronator teres:
   a. Arises by two heads from the medial and lateral epicondyles of the humerus.
   b. Has the median nerve lying between its two heads.
   c. Is supplied by the median nerve.
   d. Inserts into the lower shaft and styloid process of the ulna.
   e. Is also a flexor of the elbow joint.

34. a. True   It is also supplied by the radial, median and musculocutaneous nerves.

    b. False   The elbow joint comprises the articular surfaces of the capitulum and trochlea on the lower end of the humerus, the coronoid fossa and olecranon of the ulna and the head of the radius.

    c. True   The distal radioulnar joint however does not communicate with the wrist joint.

    d. False   It encloses the head of the radius, but is not attached to it. The head of the radius remains free to rotate within the annular ligament – an essential movement in pronation and supination.

    e. True   The ulnar collateral ligament is made up of three bands – anterior, posterior and middle – and they all provide stability to the medial aspect of the elbow joint.

35. a. True   The flexor compartment consists of five superficial and three deep muscles.

    b. False   It is the muscles of the *superficial* layer which arise from the common flexor origin.

    c. False   The muscles of the deep layer are flexor digitorum profundus, flexor pollicis longus and pronator quadratus.

    d. False   Flexor carpi ulnaris is supplied by the ulnar nerve.

    e. False   Pronator teres is the first muscle in the superficial group on the radial aspect of the flexor compartment of the forearm.

36. a. False   Pronator teres does arise via two heads, but they arise from the medial epicondyle of the humerus and the upper part of the medial surface of the ulna.

    b. True   This is a distinctive feature which helps to identify the median nerve.

    c. True   This is self-evident, since it passes between its two heads.

    d. False   In order to pronate the forearm, it has to insert into the radius.

    e. True   Since its medial head arises from the lower end of the humerus, its contraction will inevitably flex the elbow.

37. Flexor carpi radialis:
  a. Has a tendon which is easily identifiable at the wrist.
  b. Inserts into the trapezoid and trapezium.
  c. Arises from the upper shafts of both radius and ulna.
  d. Is supplied by the radial nerve.
  e. Lies between the radial artery and the median nerve at the wrist.

38. Flexor digitorum superficialis:
  a. Arises from the humerus, ulna and radius.
  b. Has four tendons which all pass below the flexor retinaculum.
  c. Is supplied entirely by the median nerve.
  d. Inserts by means of each of its four tendons into the sides of the middle phalanges of the index, middle, ring and little fingers.
  e. Flexes the distal interphalangeal joints of the index, middle, ring and little fingers.

39. Palmaris longus:
  a. Is a powerful flexor of the wrist joint.
  b. Is absent in about 10% of individuals.
  c. Arises from the medial epicondyle.
  d. Inserts into the lunate and capitate.
  e. Is supplied by the median nerve.

37. a. True Feel your own!
  b. False It inserts into the base of the thumb and index metacarpals.
  c. False It arises from the common flexor origin.
  d. False Do not be fooled by the name. It lies in the flexor compartment and is therefore supplied by the median nerve.
  e. True The artery is lateral and the nerve medial to its tendon at the wrist.

38. a. True It arises from the common flexor origin on the lower end of the humerus, medial border of the ulna and the anterior surface of the radius.
  b. True The middle two tendons lie above the tendons of the little and index fingers.
  c. True It is flexor digitorum profundus which is partially innervated by the ulnar nerve.
  d. True Each of the tendons of flexor digitorum superficialis divides into two halves which embrace the corresponding tendon of flexor digitorum profundus and insert into the sides of the middle phalanx.
  e. False It is obvious from the fact that it inserts into the middle phalanges that it cannot flex the distal interphalangeal joints. It is flexor digitorum profundus which performs that movement.

39. a. False It is a very small and weak muscle and its contraction has minimal effect.
  b. True It is believed to be a muscle which is disappearing in the human race.
  c. True It is one of the flexors in the forearm and therefore arises from the common flexor origin.
  d. False It inserts into the palmar aponeurosis.
  e. True Most of the flexors in the forearm are supplied by the median nerve. The exceptions are flexor carpi ulnaris which is supplied by the ulnar nerve and flexor digitorum profundus which is supplied by both the median and the ulnar nerves.

40. Flexor carpi ulnaris:
 a. Arises from the upper part of the shaft of the ulna.
 b. Inserts into the hook of the hamate.
 c. Is supplied by the ulnar nerve.
 d. Acts with extensor carpi ulnaris to (ulnar) adduct the wrist.
 e. Has the ulnar nerve passing between its two heads.

41. The anatomical snuffbox:
 a. Overlies the scaphoid.
 b. Contains the radial artery.
 c. Is delineated by extensor pollicis longus above, and by the two tendons of extensor pollicis brevis and flexor pollicis longus below.
 d. Also overlies the styloid process of the radius, the trapezium and the base of the thumb metacarpal.
 e. Has its skin supplied by the radial nerve.

40. a. True   It also takes origin from the common flexor origin
(the medial epicondyle) and the medial border of
the olecranon.
   b. False It inserts into the pisiform.
   c. True   This is obvious from its name and position.
   d. True   This is probably more important than its function
as a flexor of the wrist.
   e. True   The ulnar nerve then comes to lie between flexor
digitorum profundus and superficialis.

41. a. True   This is of utmost clinical importance, as it is the
site which must be examined for tenderness in
suspected fractures of the scaphoid.
   b. True   The radial artery passes from the flexor aspect of
the distal forearm into the anatomical snuffbox to
emerge in the palm, forming the deep palmar arch.
The snuffbox also contains the superficial branch of
the radial nerve.
   c. False The lower border of the anatomical snuffbox is
formed by the tendons of extensor pollicis brevis
and *abductor* pollicis longus. The tendon of flexor
pollicis longus lies in the flexor aspect of the
forearm and passes underneath the flexor
retinaculum.
   d. True   These are the other bony structures which can be
palpated in the anatomical snuffbox.
   e. True   The area of skin which is supplied exclusively by
the radial nerve is usually said to overlie the web
between the thumb and the index finger. This skin,
overlying the anatomical snuffbox, however, is also
supplied by the superficial branch of the radial
nerve.

42. Flexor digitorum profundus:
   a. Has four tendons which give origin to the interossei.
   b. Has four tendons, each of which lies in a synovial sheath which also contains the tendon of the superficial flexor.
   c. Inserts via its four tendons into the distal phalanges of the index, middle, ring and little fingers.
   d. Arises from the humerus, ulna and interosseous membrane.
   e. Is able to contract most forcefully when the wrist is fully flexed.

43. The cubital fossa:
   a. Is a diamond-shaped area on the anterior aspect of the upper limb at the level of the elbow joint.
   b. Is delineated inferiorly by brachioradialis and the bicipital tendon.
   c. Contains the brachial artery which lies medial to the median nerve.
   d. Has its floor formed by pronator quadratus.
   e. Contains the radial nerve.

42. a. False It is the *lumbricals* which arise from the tendons of flexor digitorum profundus. The interossei arise from the metacarpals.

    b. True The flexor sheaths contain the tendons of flexor digitorum profundus and superficialis.

    c. True The tendons of flexor digitorum profundus insert into the terminal phalanges, and the tendons of flexor digitorum superficialis insert into the middle phalanges.

    d. False Flexor digitorum profundus does not arise from the lower humerus. It only takes origin from the olecranon, shaft of the ulna and the interosseous membrane.

    e. False This is a fact which is made use of in self-defence classes. When attacked by an assailant with a knife, forcibly flexing his (or her) wrist will make the assailant drop the knife as the grip is weakened!

43. a. False The cubital fossa is triangular in shape. It is the popliteal fossa which is diamond-shaped.

    b. False The cubital fossa is bordered by brachioradialis, pronator teres and a line joining the two epicondyles of the humerus. The bicipital tendon lies within the cubital fossa.

    c. False The median nerve is the most medial structure among the contents of the cubital fossa.

    d. False Pronator quadratus lies in the distal forearm. The floor of the cubital fossa is formed mainly by brachialis.

    e. True Both the radial nerve and its posterior interosseous branch lie in the lateral part of the cubital fossa.

44. Flexor pollicis longus:
  a. Is one of the three outcropping muscles of the forearm.
  b. Arises from the radius and the interosseous membrane.
  c. Has a tendon which crosses over the flexor retinaculum.
  d. Inserts into the distal phalanx of the thumb.
  e. Is innervated via the median nerve.

45. In the forearm:
  a. The anterior interosseous nerve arises from the ulnar nerve.
  b. The posterior interosseous nerve arises from the radial nerve.
  c. The common interosseous artery arises directly from the brachial artery.
  d. Pronator quadratus lies superficial to the tendons of flexor digitorum profundus.
  e. The flexor compartment receives most of its blood supply from the anterior interosseous artery.

44. a. False The three outcropping muscles of the forearm all lie on the extensor surface of the forearm and move the thumb. They are extensor pollicis longus and brevis and abductor pollicis longus. They are called 'outcropping' because they cross over brachioradialis and extensor carpi radialis longus and brevis to reach their insertions.

   b. True Some fibres also take origin from the ulna.

   c. False No tendon crosses over the flexor retinaculum. The tendon of flexor pollicis longus is one of the 10 tendons which lie in the carpal tunnel. The others are the eight tendons of flexor digitorum superficialis and profundus, and the tendon of flexor carpi radialis.

   d. True It therefore flexes the thumb at its interphalangeal joint.

   e. True The three muscles of the thenar eminence and flexor pollicis longus are all innervated via the median nerve. Flexor pollicis longus receives its innervation via the anterior interosseous branch of the median nerve.

45. a. False The anterior interosseous nerve arises from the median nerve.

   b. True It supplies most of the muscles in the extensor compartment of the forearm.

   c. False It arises from the ulnar artery and it divides into anterior and posterior interosseous arteries.

   d. False Pronator quadratus lies deep in the flexor compartment of the forearm, and the tendons of flexor digitorum profundus lie on it.

   e. True The anterior interosseous artery is the much larger of the two branches of the common interosseous artery and is the main source of blood to the flexor compartment of the forearm.

46. In the posterior compartment of the forearm:
   a. Brachioradialis arises from the humerus and inserts into the distal radius.
   b. Supinator arises in two parts, with the radial nerve passing between its two components.
   c. The blood supply is derived mainly from the ulnar artery.
   d. The tendon of extensor digiti minimi is usually double.
   e. All the muscles arise from the common extensor origin.

47. In the posterior compartment of the forearm:
   a. Brachioradialis overlies the radial nerve and artery.
   b. Extensor carpi radialis longus arises from the lateral supracondylar ridge of the humerus.
   c. Extensor carpi radialis brevis inserts into the dorsal aspect of the trapezium and scaphoid.
   d. Extensor digitorum is supplied by the ulnar nerve.
   e. Supinator is the most powerful muscle producing supination.

46. a. True   It is therefore a flexor of the elbow.
   b. False   Supinator does arise in two parts – one from the upper part of the ulna, and the other from the lateral epicondyle of the humerus, but it is the *posterior interosseous nerve* and not the radial which passes between its two parts.
   c. True   The arteries which supply the posterior compartment of the forearm are the posterior and anterior interosseous arteries. They both arise from the common interosseous artery, which is a branch of the ulnar.
   d. True   It is subsequently joined by the slip from extensor digitorum to the little finger, and they are all enclosed in a single synovial sheath.
   e. False   The common extensor origin gives rise to the fused tendons of extensor carpi radialis brevis, extensor digitorum, extensor digiti minimi and extensor carpi ulnaris. The origin of some of the other muscles in the posterior compartment of the forearm will be dealt with shortly.

47. a. True   This is the best place to locate the radial nerve when asked to do so in a viva – under brachioradialis.
   b. True   This is the origin of brachioradialis and extensor carpi radialis longus.
   c. False   It inserts into the base of the third metacarpal.
   d. False   It is supplied by the posterior interosseous nerve, which is a branch of the radial nerve. It is the nerve of the posterior compartment of the forearm and supplies most of the muscles within it.
   e. False   The most powerful supinator is biceps brachii.

48. The outcropping muscles:
 a. Include abductor pollicis brevis, which is innervated by the posterior interosseous nerve.
 b. Include extensor pollicis brevis, which inserts into the base of the distal phalanx.
 c. Cross over the tendons of brachialis, extensor carpi radialis longus and extensor indicis.
 d. Include extensor pollicis longus, which forms the upper border of the anatomical snuffbox.
 e. Are all supplied by the posterior interosseous nerve, which has a root value of $C_{5,6}$.

49. The extensor retinaculum:
 a. Is attached to the distal radius and the styloid process of the ulna.
 b. Lies transversely across the distal part of the extensor surface of the forearm.
 c. Has extensor pollicis longus and brevis passing underneath it within a single common synovial sheath.
 d. Has the tendons of extensor carpi radialis longus and brevis and extensor carpi ulnaris crossing over it to reach their insertions.
 e. Has the four tendons of extensor digitorum and the tendon of extensor indicis passing underneath it within a common synovial sheath.

48. a. False Abductor pollicis brevis is one of the thenar
muscles and not one of the outcropping muscles.
It is supplied by the recurrent branch of the median
nerve.

    b. False It is the tendon of extensor pollicis *longus* which
inserts into the base of the distal phalanx. The
tendon of extensor pollicis brevis inserts into the
base of the *proximal* phalanx. This can logically be
deduced from their names.

    c. False They cross over *brachioradialis*, extensor carpi
radialis longus *and brevis*. Extensor indicis lies on
the ulnar aspect of the outcropping muscles and is
therefore not crossed by them.

    d. True The lower border is formed by the other two
outcropping muscles – extensor pollicis brevis and
abductor pollicis longus.

    e. False They *are* all supplied by the posterior interosseous
nerve; its root value however is $C_{7,8}$.

49. a. False It is attached to the distal radius and the pisiform
and triquetral bones. If it were attached to both the
radius and ulna, it would impede pronation and
supination.

    b. False The flexor retinaculum lies transversely, whereas the
extensor retinaculum lies obliquely, being attached
more proximally on the radial aspect.

    c. False The two extensor tendons of the thumb delineate the
borders of the anatomical snuffbox, and are some
distance away from each other. They therefore pass
under the extensor retinaculum lying within their
own separate synovial sheaths. Extensor pollicis
brevis may sometimes share its synovial sheath with
abductor pollicis longus.

    d. False All the extensor tendons pass underneath the
extensor retinaculum, to prevent 'bow-stringing'
when their muscles contract.

    e. True The tendon of extensor digiti minimi however
usually has its own separate synovial sheath.

50. The thenar eminence:
   a.   Is made of three muscles which move the thumb – adductor pollicis, flexor pollicis brevis and opponens pollicis.
   b.   Includes opponens pollicis which lies deep to the other two muscles of the thenar eminence.
   c.   Includes opponens pollicis which arises from the flexor retinaculum and the trapezium and inserts into the thumb metacarpal.
   d.   Is made up of three muscles, and they all contain fibres which have taken origin from the flexor retinaculum.
   e.   Is made up of three muscles which are all innervated by the superficial branch of the median nerve and are therefore unaffected in carpal tunnel syndrome.

51. The hypothenar muscles:
   a.   Are all innervated by the median nerve.
   b.   Are abductor, flexor and opponens digiti minimi.
   c.   All have fibres which take origin from the flexor retinaculum.
   d.   Strengthen the grip.
   e.   Include opponens digiti minimi which inserts into the proximal phalanx of the little finger.

50. a. False Adductor pollicis is a muscle which lies in a much
deeper plane. The muscles which make up the
thenar eminence are *abductor pollicis brevis*, flexor
pollicis brevis and opponens pollicis.
 b. True It is the deepest of the three thenar muscles.
 c. True Its contraction will therefore oppose the thumb.
 d. True Abductor pollicis brevis arises from the flexor
retinaculum and the scaphoid, whereas flexor
pollicis brevis and opponens pollicis take origin
from the flexor retinaculum and the trapezium.
 e. False The superficial branch of the median nerve supplies
the skin overlying the thenar eminence, which is
unaffected in carpal tunnel syndrome. The muscles
themselves however are usually innervated by a
branch from the median nerve itself after it has
passed through the carpal tunnel. This accounts for
the atrophy of the thenar muscles which often
accompanies long-standing carpal tunnel syndrome.

51. a. False They are all innervated by a branch of the ulnar
nerve.
 b. True They are similar in name and function to the
muscles of the thenar eminence (though they
obviously move the little finger and not the thumb).
 c. True This is another feature which they have in common
with the muscles of the thenar eminence. Abductor
digiti minimi arises from the flexor retinaculum and
the pisiform, flexor digiti minimi arises from the
flexor retinaculum, and opponens digiti minimi
arises from the flexor retinaculum and the hook of
the hamate.
 d. True This is their main function.
 e. False In order to oppose the little finger it has to insert
into the fifth metacarpal. If it were inserted into the
proximal phalanx, its contraction would flex the
little finger.

52. Adductor pollicis:
   a. Arises via two heads.
   b. Has a transverse head which arises from the third metacarpal and inserts into the proximal phalanx of the thumb.
   c. Has an oblique head which arises from the thumb metacarpal and inserts into the proximal phalanx of the thumb.
   d. Is innervated by the median nerve.
   e. Assists in opposition and flexion of the thumb.

53. The blood supply of the hand:
   a. Includes the princeps pollicis artery and the arteria radialis indicis, both of which arise from the radial artery.
   b. Includes the deep palmar arch which is deeper and more proximal than the superficial palmar arch.
   c. Is derived in part from the radial artery which reaches the palm by passing through the anatomical snuffbox, between the two heads of the first dorsal interosseous muscle and the transverse and oblique heads of adductor pollicis.
   d. Includes the superficial palmar arch which is mainly derived from the ulnar artery.
   e. Includes the deep palmar arch which is often not a complete arch.

52. a. True It is similar in many respects to adductor hallucis in the sole of the foot.

b. True It also inserts into the tendon of extensor pollicis longus and the ulnar sesamoid.

c. False Such a muscle would be a flexor of the thumb. The oblique head of adductor pollicis arises from the second and third metacarpals and from the trapezoid and capitate. It inserts into the ulnar sesamoid.

d. False It is not a thenar muscle. It is classified as one of the small muscles of the hand and is innervated by the deep branch of the ulnar nerve.

e. False It is, as its name implies, merely an adductor of the thumb, assisting in approximating the thumb to the index finger.

53. a. True They arise from the radial artery before it forms the deep palmar arch.

b. True The deep palmar arch overlies the bases of the metacarpals, whereas the superficial palmar arch lies just underneath the palmar aponeurosis, usually at the level of the proximal transverse palmar crease.

c. True Having passed between the two heads of adductor pollicis, the radial artery then forms the deep palmar arch.

d. True The superficial palmar arch is mainly derived from the ulnar artery and the deep palmar arch is mainly derived from the radial.

e. False It is the *superficial* palmar arch which is often incomplete. The deep palmar arch is usually a complete arch and anastomoses at its ulnar end with the deep branch of the ulnar artery.

54. The interossei:
a.   Are all innervated by the median nerve.
b.   Are divided into palmar and dorsal, the former being the larger and more powerful.
c.   Include the palmar interossei which adduct the fingers.
d.   Include the dorsal interossei which all arise via two heads.

55. The flexor tendons of the fingers:
a.   Lie within a common synovial sheath which envelops both the superficial and deep flexor tendons of each finger.
b.   Include the tendons of flexor digitorum superficialis which insert distal to the tendons of flexor digitorum profundus.
c.   Include the tendons of flexor digitorum superficialis which divide into two elements and pass behind the deep tendons.
d.   Have long and short vinculae which are vascular synovial folds.
e.   Receive their blood supply through the vinculae.

54. a. False All the interossei are usually innervated by the ulnar nerve.
　　b. False It is the other way round. The dorsal interossei are much larger than the palmar interossei and can therefore be seen from the palmar aspect.
　　c. True PAD and DAB is the way to remember this. The **P**almar interossei **AD**duct, whereas the **D**orsal interossei **AB**duct. The axis about which these movements occur is the middle finger.
　　d. True Each dorsal interosseous muscle arises via two heads, one from each metacarpal bordering the interosseous space.

55. a. True The superficial and deep flexor tendons of each finger are enclosed within one common synovial sheath.
　　b. False The superficial tendons insert into the middle phalanx whereas the deep tendons insert into the distal phalanx.
　　c. True At this point the profundus tendon becomes superficial to the two parts of the superficialis tendon.
　　d. True Each of the superficial and deep tendons has a short and long vinculum.
　　e. True The flexor tendons receive their blood supply through the long vinculae. Some authorities claim that the short vinculae also provide a blood supply to the flexor tendons.

56. The extensor expansions:
   a. Divide into three parts distally.
   b. Are made up of the extensor tendon, the lumbricals and the interossei.
   c. Contribute to flexion of the metacarpophalangeal joint.
   d. Insert into the proximal, middle and distal phalanges.
   e. Are affected in radial nerve injuries, but not in injuries of the median or ulnar nerves.

57. The median nerve:
   a. Has a root value of C_{5-7}.
   b. Provides innervation to the shoulder joint.
   c. Is sensory to the palmar aspect of the little, ring and middle fingers and half the index finger.
   d. Supplies pronator quadratus.
   e. Lies deep to the tendons of flexor digitorum superficialis at the wrist.

56. a. True The central slip inserts into the dorsal aspect of the base of the middle phalanx, whereas the two lateral slips insert into the dorsal aspect of the base of the terminal phalanx.

  b. True The lumbricals and interossei insert into the sides of the extensor tendons.

  c. True This is achieved by contraction of the dorsal and palmar interossei together. Their abductor and adductor effects cancel each other out, and they pull down the fingers by means of their insertion into the dorsal expansion, thus flexing the metacarpophalangeal joint.

  d. False They do not insert into the proximal phalanges. The latter receive the attachments of the palmar aponeurosis.

  e. False The posterior interosseous branch of the radial nerve supplies extensor digitorum, extensor indicis and extensor digiti minimi. The ulnar nerve usually supplies all the interossei, and the median and ulnar nerves supply the lumbricals. Injury to any of these three nerves will affect the action of the dorsal expansion.

57. a. False The median nerve innervates some of the small muscles of the hand, therefore it must contain T_1 fibres. Its root value is $C_{6-8} T_1$.

  b. False It does not supply the muscles which move the shoulder joint and therefore does not supply it.

  c. False It is sensory to the palmar aspect of the *radial* three-and-a-half fingers, i.e. the thumb, index and middle fingers and half the ring finger. It also innervates their nail beds.

  d. True Both pronators are supplied by the median nerve, the quadratus via the anterior interosseous branch and pronator teres from the trunk of the nerve itself.

  e. False The median nerve lies between the tendons of flexor carpi radialis and palmaris longus at the level of the wrist. It lies in the same plane as the tendons of flexor digitorum superficialis, not deep to them.

58. The ulnar nerve:
    a.   Has a root value of C_{5-7}.
    b.   Passes just medial to the pisiform bone.
    c.   Carries nerve fibres which supply the elbow joint.
    d.   Supplies skin on both the palmar and dorsal aspects of the hand.
    e.   Supplies palmaris brevis.

59. The clavicle:
    a.   Is crossed by the supraclavicular nerves.
    b.   Has two articular surfaces on its medial end.
    c.   Provides attachment to both trapezius and deltoid.
    d.   Is attached to the scapula by means of the acromioclavicular and the coracoclavicular ligaments.
    e.   Is the first bone which is formed in the fetal skeleton.

58. a. False Again, since the ulnar nerve is the main nerve
supplying the small muscles of the hand, it must
have T_1 fibres (see previous question). The root
value of the ulnar nerve is $C_{7,8} T_1$.

   b. True It can be rolled against the hook of the hamate,
producing an unpleasant sensation.

   c. True It usually supplies flexor carpi ulnaris which arises
above the elbow, and therefore can be considered a
mover of that joint. So, according to Hilton's law,
the elbow joint receives innervation from the ulnar
nerve – the nerve which supplies the muscle which
moves that joint.

   d. True It usually supplies the skin on palmar and dorsal
aspects of the little and half the ring fingers and the
corresponding amount of the skin of the hand.

   e. True It is the only muscle supplied by the superficial
branch of the ulnar which is mainly cutaneous.

59. a. True This is obvious from their name. They sometimes
even pass through it!

   b. True One articulates with the manubrium sterni, and the
second, which lies on the inferior aspect of the
medial end of the clavicle, articulates with the first
costal cartilage.

   c. True Deltoid arises from the lateral third of the clavicle,
the lateral part of the acromion process and the
spine of the scapula. Trapezius inserts into the
posterior aspect of the lateral third of the clavicle,
the medial part of the acromion process and the
spine of the scapula.

   d. True As their names indicate, they attach the clavicle to
the acromion process and the coracoid process of
the scapula respectively. Of the two, the latter is by
far the stronger, and has two components – the
conoid and trapezoid ligaments.

   e. True It starts to form in the fifth week of intrauterine
life.

60. The scapula:
  a. Has a spine on its dorsal surface which delineates the upper limit for the origin of the fibres of subscapularis.
  b. Has the digitations of serratus anterior inserting into its lateral border.
  c. Has the coracoid process projecting forwards as the lateral projection of the spine of the scapula.
  d. Gives attachment to both heads of biceps brachii.
  e. Has the coracoid process which provides attachment to three muscles and three ligaments.

61. The humerus:
  a. Gives origin to all three heads of triceps.
  b. Carries the capitulum on its lower end which articulates with the coronoid process of the ulna.
  c. Carries on its lower end the trochlea which has an articular surface covering both its anterior and posterior aspects.
  d. Carries a medial supracondylar ridge which gives origin to pronator teres.
  e. Has the ulnar nerve passing behind its lateral epicondyle.

60. a. False Subscapularis arises from the *ventral* surface of the scapula.

    b. False The digitations of serratus anterior insert into the *medial* border and inferior angle of the scapula.

    c. False It is the *acromion* process which is the terminal lateral projection of the spine of the scapula.

    d. True The long head arises from just above the glenoid fossa, within the shoulder joint capsule, whereas the short head arises from the coracoid process.

    e. True The ligaments are the coracoclavicular (with its two parts – the conoid and trapezoid), the coracohumeral and the coracoacromial, and the three muscles are pectoralis minor, coracobrachialis and the short head of biceps brachii.

61. a. False If all three heads of triceps arose from the humerus, it would be unable to extend the shoulder. The medial and lateral heads arise from the humerus. The long head arises from the infraglenoid tubercle of the scapula.

    b. False The capitulum articulates with the head of the radius. The coronoid and olecranon processes of the ulna articulate with the trochlea.

    c. True This is to provide an articular area to accommodate the full range of flexion/extension at the elbow joint.

    d. True In order to pronate the forearm, pronator teres must arise from the medial aspect of the lower humerus and insert into the radius. It also takes origin from the medial epicondyle and the coronoid process of the ulna.

    e. False If you palpate just behind your *medial* epicondyle you will be able to feel your ulnar nerve.

62. The radius:
   a. Has a head which articulates with the scaphoid and lunate bones at the wrist.
   b. Has the tendon of brachioradialis inserting into the base of its styloid process.
   c. Has the tendon of biceps brachii inserting into the radial tubercle.
   d. Gives origin to the fibres of both flexor digitorum superficialis and flexor digitorum profundus.
   e. Has a number of grooves on the dorsal surface of its lower end.

63. The ulna:
   a. Has the tendon of triceps inserting into the posterior surface of the olecranon process.
   b. Carries the 'sublime' tubercle on its coronoid process, which gives origin to some of the fibres of flexor digitorum superficialis.
   c. Carries the coronoid process which receives the insertion of brachialis.
   d. Has the annular ligament attached to the anterior and posterior margins of the radial notch.
   e. Has the trochlear notch proximally which carries the articular surfaces of the olecranon and coronoid processes.

62. a. False The head of the radius lies proximally. It is held within the annular ligament which binds it to the proximal ulna. It articulates with the capitulum on the distal end of the humerus as part of the elbow joint, and with the radial notch of the ulna in the superior radioulnar joint.

   b. True It arises from the lateral aspect of the lower end of the humerus and inserts into the distal radius.

   c. False The bicipital tendon inserts into the bicipital tuberosity which lies on the inner aspect of the upper part of the shaft of the radius. The radial tubercle lies on the dorsal surface of its distal end.

   d. False The fibres of flexor digitorum profundus arise from the common flexor origin (on the humerus), the ulna and the interosseous membrane, but *not* from the radius. Flexor digitorum superficialis, however, arises from the common flexor origin, the ulna and the anterior oblique line of the radius.

   e. True They are for the various compartments of the extensor tendons as they cross beneath the extensor retinaculum.

63. a. True Contraction of the triceps will therefore extend the elbow joint.

   b. True The original name for flexor digitorum superficialis, which may still be found in some older anatomy textbooks, is sublimis.

   c. True Brachialis arises from the mid-shaft of the humerus and inserts into the coronoid process of the ulna. It is one of the flexors of the elbow joint.

   d. True It thus encircles the head of the radius and keeps it in contact with the radial notch of the ulna.

   e. True The trochlear notch is covered with hyaline cartilage and articulates with the trochlea on the lower end of the humerus.

64. Nerve injuries in the upper limb include:
- a. Damage to the entire brachial plexus which may lead to Horner's syndrome.
- b. Erb's palsy, which is a birth injury involving the upper roots and upper trunk.
- c. Klumpke's paralysis, which may also be associated with Horner's syndrome.
- d. Paraesthesia in a diamond-shaped area on the lateral aspect of the arm, 2.5 cm below the acromion following dislocation of the shoulder.
- e. Drop wrist following fractures of the shaft of the humerus.

64. a. True Sympathetic fibres arise between T_1 and L_2. The fibres destined for the pupil, the visceral part of levator palpebrae superioris and the sweat glands of the face emerge with the T_1 nerve root and can therefore be damaged in injuries involving the brachial plexus.

b. True It is the fibres arising from $C_{5,6}$ which are involved. They contribute to the fibres of the musculocutaneous and axillary nerves, therefore shoulder abduction, elbow flexion and supination are abolished. The lateral rotators of the shoulder are also affected. The upper limb is therefore held in medial rotation with the elbow extended and the palm facing backwards. This position has been likened to the position in which the arm is held when soliciting a furtive tip.

c. True Klumpke's paralysis can occur in breech deliveries when the arm remains above the head during delivery. It is caused by injury to the C_8T_1 roots and it is mainly the small muscles of the hand which are affected but, due to injury of the T_1 nerve root, Horner's syndrome may also occur.

d. True Dislocation of the shoulder may lead to injury to the axillary nerve. The inability actively to abduct the shoulder due to paralysis of the deltoid may be misinterpreted as reluctance to move the dislocated shoulder because of the pain, and therefore the presence or absence of paraesthesia in this area should always be elicited following dislocation of the shoulder.

e. True The radial nerve can be injured in fractures involving the shaft of the humerus. This leads to inability to extend the wrist as it is the posterior interosseous branch of the radial nerve which supplies the extensors of the wrist.

65. In the upper limb:
   a.   Injuries of the ulnar nerve will lead to clawing of the hand.
   b.   Injuries of the median nerve cause what is described as ape hand.
   c.   The clawing which can occur after a supracondylar fracture is usually more severe than the clawing caused by damage to the T_1 nerve root.
   d.   Injuries of the ulnar nerve lead to loss of opposition of the thumb.
   e.   Injury to the ulnar nerve will give the hands a thin, bony appearance.

65. a. True This is caused by paralysis of the interossei and the lumbricals innervated by the ulnar nerve (usually the two on the ulnar side). The clawing is therefore more pronounced in the little and ring fingers.

   b. True Injuries of the median nerve lead to atrophy of the muscles of the thenar eminence. The presence of these muscles that move the thumb is the main difference between the human and simian hand. A human hand with a long-standing median nerve injury has a flattened thenar eminence which is similar to the hand of an ape.

   c. False Clawing of the hand after a supracondylar fracture is due to ulnar nerve injury. In this case, the lumbricals supplied by the median nerve (usually the two radial ones) are unaffected, and the clawing would be less severe than that caused by a T_1 nerve root injury, as in that case all the small muscles of the hand would be affected.

   d. False Opponens pollicis is usually supplied by the median nerve, and is therefore unaffected in ulnar nerve injuries.

   e. True This is due to wasting of the interossei.

Lower limb

1. **The venous drainage of the lower limb:**
   a. Includes the great (or long) saphenous vein which runs up the medial aspect of the lower limb just behind the medial malleolus.
   b. Includes the small (or short) saphenous vein which opens into the popliteal vein which lies deep to the tibial nerve.
   c. Consists of numerous channels connecting the deep and superficial veins in which the blood flows from the deep to the superficial veins.
   d. Drains into the femoral vein which lies medial to the femoral artery at the level of the inguinal ligament.
   e. The great (or long) saphenous vein is a common site for varicosities as it contains no valves.

2. **The arches of the foot:**
   a. Include the medial longitudinal arch which consists of the calcaneus, talus, the medial and intermediate cuneiform and the first two metatarsals.
   b. Include the lateral longitudinal arch which consists of the calcaneus, navicular, cuboid and the lateral two metatarsals.
   c. Include the transverse arch which is only half an arch and is completed by the transverse arch of the other foot.
   d. Are supported by the tendon of peroneus longus which is inserted into the base of the fifth metatarsal and the cuboid bone.
   e. Are also supported by the ligaments of the foot which include the short and long plantar ligaments.

1. a. False The great saphenous vein runs up the medial aspect
            of the lower limb passing just *anterior to* the medial
            malleolus. This is considered one of the most
            clinically important anatomical facts as it can be
            cannulated blindly, even in shocked patients.
    b. True   This is an unusual situation as the nerve lies
            superficial to the vein in this area.
    c. False The venous blood flows from the superficial to the
            deep veins. It only flows in the reverse direction
            when there is a blockage in the deep veins, and this
            leads to varices.
    d. True   This is a useful anatomical fact to know when
            attempting to obtain a sample of venous blood
            from the femoral vein. The needle should be
            inserted just medial to the pulsations of the femoral
            artery.
    e. False It usually has over a dozen valves. Varicosities are
            usually associated with incompetence of these
            valves.

2. a. False The medial longitudinal arch consists of the
            calcaneus, talus, navicular, the three cuneiforms
            and their metatarsals.
    b. False The navicular bone is on the medial aspect of the
            foot. The lateral longitudinal arch consists of the
            calcaneus, cuboid and the lateral two metatarsals.
    c. True   It consists of the bases of the five metatarsals, the
            cuboid and the three cuneiforms.
    d. False The tendon of peroneus longus does support the
            arches of the foot. However, it inserts into the base
            of the first metatarsal and the medial cuneiform.
    e. True   Other ligaments of the foot also play a role in
            supporting the arches of the foot. These include the
            spring ligament, the dorsal, plantar and
            interosseous ligaments between the small bones of
            the forefoot, and the plantar aponeurosis.

3. **In the foot:**
   a. The dorsalis pedis artery pulsations can be felt in all normal individuals between the tendon of tibialis anterior and the tendon of extensor hallucis longus.
   b. The dorsalis pedis artery is a direct continuation of the anterior tibial artery.
   c. The posterior tibial artery runs between the tendons of flexor digitorum longus and flexor hallucis longus behind the medial malleolus.
   d. The posterior tibial nerve divides into medial and lateral plantar nerves which carry sensation from the sole of the foot in a manner similar to the way the ulnar and median nerves carry sensation from the palm of the hand.
   e. The tendon of tibialis posterior lies posterior to the tendons of flexor digitorum longus and flexor hallucis longus at the level of the medial malleolus.

4. **In the foot:**
   a. The abductor hallucis is supplied by the medial plantar nerve.
   b. The plantar aponeurosis is attached to the medial and lateral tubercles of the calcaneum and the inferior surface of the talus.
   c. The two lateral dorsal and plantar interossei are supplied by the lateral plantar nerve.
   d. There are a total of seven interossei – three plantar and four dorsal.
   e. The plantar interossei abduct the second, third and fourth toes.

3. a. False These are the correct anatomical landmarks for the dorsalis pedis artery. However, the pulse may be absent in a small percentage of normal individuals, so its absence may not indicate blockage of the vessel.

b. True The anterior tibial artery becomes the dorsalis pedis artery when it reaches the dorsum of the foot.

c. True See mnemonic in e.

d. True The lateral plantar nerve corresponds to the ulnar nerve and supplies the lateral one-and-a-half toes, whereas the medial plantar nerve corresponds to the median nerve, which supplies the medial three-and-a-half toes.

e. False A useful mnemonic to remember the relations of the tendons passing behind the medial malleolus is: Tom, Dick and Harry – Tibialis posterior, flexor Digitorum longus and flexor Hallucis longus. An even better mnemonic is: The Doctors Are Never Happy – Tibialis posterior, flexor Digitorum longus, posterior tibial Artery, Nerve, vein, flexor Hallucis longus, as it contains the reminder that the artery, nerve and vein also lie posterior to the medial malleolus, between the tendons of flexor digitorum longus and flexor hallucis longus. Note, however, that the vein usually lies between the nerve and the artery.

4. a. True The medial plantar nerve supplies the abductor hallucis, the flexor hallucis brevis, the flexor digitorum brevis and the first lumbrical.

b. False It arises only from the calcaneum.

c. True All the interossei are supplied by the lateral plantar nerve.

d. True There are only three plantar interossei, as the first plantar interosseous muscle has merged into the adductor hallucis.

e. False The plantar interossei adduct and the dorsal interossei abduct. As in the hand, the mnemonics are PAD – Plantars ADduct – and DAB – Dorsals ABduct. Remember that the interossei also stabilize the metatarsophalangeal and interphalangeal joints during walking.

5. The ligaments of the foot include:
a. The long plantar ligament which lies deep to the short plantar ligament.
b. The long plantar ligament which extends from the plantar surface of the calcaneus to the cuboid and the bases of the third, fourth and fifth metatarsals.
c. The spring ligament (the plantar calcaneonavicular ligament) which is a strong band passing from the sustentaculum tali to the navicular bone.
d. The long plantar ligament which forms a tunnel for the peroneus brevis tendon as it passes to its insertion.
e. The short plantar ligament, which is also called the plantar calcaneocuboid.

6. The muscles of the anterior compartment of the thigh include:
a. The rectus femoris, which arises from the pubis by two heads.
b. The vastus lateralis whose lower fibres insert into the patella in an almost horizontal manner, thus helping to prevent medial dislocation of the patella.
c. Pectineus, which is sometimes innervated by a branch of the obturator nerve.
d. Iliacus and psoas major, which are powerful flexors and lateral rotators of the hip joint.
e. Iliacus and psoas major, which insert via a common tendon into the greater trochanter of the femur.

7. The muscles of the posterior compartment of the thigh:
a. Are separated from the anterior compartment by the lateral intermuscular septum, but are continuous with the adductor compartment.
b. Include biceps femoris whose tendon is a distinctive landmark on the medial aspect of the popliteal fossa.
c. All arise from the ischial tuberosity.
d. Are all supplied by branches of the sciatic nerve.
e. Are flexors of the knee joint and extensors of the hip.

5. a. False It is the short plantar ligament which lies deep to the long plantar ligament.
   b. True It plays a role in supporting the arches of the foot.
   c. True The sustentaculum tali is a projection from the calcaneus. It is Latin for 'support of the talus'.
   d. False The peroneus brevis inserts into the base of the fifth metatarsal. It is the peroneus longus which passes through the tunnel underneath the long plantar ligament.
   e. True The short plantar ligament extends from the plantar surface of the calcaneus to the cuboid, hence its other name.

6. a. False The rectus femoris does arise by two heads – a straight head from the anterior inferior iliac spine, and a reflected head from the ilium, just above the acetabulum. Neither head arises from the pubis.
   b. False It is the vastus *medialis* whose lower fibres insert in an almost horizontal manner and play a role in preventing *lateral* dislocation of the patella.
   c. True It can be innervated by the femoral nerve, the obturator nerve or both. This reflects its double origin from the flexor (adductor) and extensor (anterior) compartment.
   d. False Iliacus and psoas major are powerful flexors and *medial* rotators of the hip joint.
   e. False Iliacus and psoas major insert via a common tendon into and just below the *lesser* trochanter of the femur.

7. a. True This is due to the presence of adductor magnus which consists of fused flexor and adductor components.
   b. False The tendon of biceps femoris is a distinctive landmark on the *lateral* aspect of the popliteal fossa.
   c. False Semimembranosus, semitendinosus and the long head of biceps femoris arise from the ischial tuberosity. The short head of biceps, however, arises from the back of the femur.
   d. True The hamstring portion of adductor magnus is supplied by the sciatic nerve. Its adductor portion is supplied by the obturator nerve.
   e. True They contract rhythmically during walking and running.

8. The muscles of the medial compartment of the thigh:
   a. Are supplied by the profunda femoris and obturator arteries.
   b. Are supplied by branches of the femoral and obturator nerves.
   c. Include adductor magnus which has a hiatus between its adductor and hamstring components through which the sciatic nerve passes.
   d. Include adductor longus which arises from the body of the pubis by a strong round tendon which may be ossified.
   e. Include adductor brevis which lies superficial to adductor longus.

9. The medial aspect of the upper tibia:
   a. Is the site of insertion of three muscles – sartorius, gracilis and biceps femoris.
   b. Receives the sartorius muscle which is innervated by the obturator nerve.
   c. Receives the gracilis muscle which is one of the adductors of the thigh.
   d. Is the site of the bursa which separates the three tendons.
   e. Receives three muscles, each of which is supplied by a different nerve.

8. a. True   The profunda femoris arises from the femoral artery, and the obturator artery is one of the branches of the anterior division of the internal iliac artery.

  b. False   They are all supplied by the obturator nerve except the hamstring portion of adductor magnus which is also supplied by a branch of the sciatic nerve.

  c. False   It is the femoral artery and vein which pass through the hiatus separating the two components of the adductor magnus.

  d. True   This is the 'rider's bone' which is easily palpable on the medial aspect of the thigh. It becomes more noticeable when the thigh is adducted against resistance.

  e. False   It lies deep to pectineus and adductor longus. The anterior and posterior divisions of the obturator nerve pass superficial and deep to the adductor brevis muscle respectively.

9. a. False   It is, from lateral to medial, sartorius, gracilis and semitendinosus which insert into the medial aspect of the upper end of the tibia. The well-known mnemonic giving the sequence of their insertion is: **S**ay **G**race **B**efore **T**ea – **S**artorius, **G**racilis, **B**ursa, semi**T**endinosus.

  b. False   Sartorius is innervated by the femoral nerve and is so named for its ability to flex and medially rotate the leg, to draw the leg into the position taken up by tailors who sat cross-legged during their work (*sartorius*, a tailor: Latin). Sartorius has the distinction of being the longest muscle in the body.

  c. True   The others are adductor longus, brevis and magnus.

  d. True   This is the bursa anserina, which has been likened to a goose's foot.

  e. True   Sartorius is innervated by the femoral nerve, gracilis by the obturator and semitendinosus by the sciatic. Another point of interest is that each muscle arises from a different bone. Sartorius arises from the ilium, gracilis from the pubis and semitendinosus from the ischium.

10. The knee joint:
   a. Is a hinge joint made up of the articulations between the femur, tibia and fibula.
   b. Includes the tendon of popliteus which perforates the capsule posteriorly and attaches to the medial meniscus.
   c. Has medial and lateral patellar retinaculae which are attached to the sides of the patella and are expansions from vasti medialis and lateralis respectively.
   d. Has the anterior cruciate ligament which arises from the posterior intercondylar area on the superior aspect of the tibia.
   e. Contains two semilunar cartilages, the medial one being larger and more liable for injury.

11. The iliotibial tract:
   a. Is a thickening of fascia lata on the lateral aspect of the thigh.
   b. Receives the insertion of most of the fibres of gluteus maximus.
   c. Helps maintain the erect posture by keeping the knee extended.
   d. Inserts into the head of the fibula and the lateral aspect of the tibia.
   e. Receives the insertion of tensor fascia lata, which is supplied by the superior gluteal nerve.

10. a. False The articulations are between the femoral and tibial condyles, and between the patella and the patellar surface of the femur. There is no fibular involvement.

 b. False The tendon of popliteus is attached to the lateral margin of the lateral meniscus, and this is one of the reasons why the lateral meniscus is less commonly injured than the medial meniscus. It is said that the lateral meniscus is pulled out of harm's way by contraction of popliteus.

 c. True They are said to play a role in stabilizing the position of the patella and thus preventing its dislocation.

 d. False The anterior and posterior cruciate ligaments are named according to the position to which they are attached on the superior surface of the tibia. The function of the two cruciate ligaments is to maintain the approximation between the femur and the tibia. The anterior cruciate ligament forms the axis around which the knee medially rotates in the last few degrees of extension. The posterior cruciate prevents anterior dislocation of the femur from the tibial plateau.

 e. True This injury is usually caused by internal rotation of the femur on the fixed weight-bearing tibia with the knee partially flexed – an injury commonly seen in football players.

11. a. True The fascia lata encloses all the thigh. The iliotibial tract is the thickened fascia on the lateral aspect.

 b. True It is said to receive three-quarters of the fibres of gluteus maximus which insert in common with the fibres of tensor fascia lata.

 c. True This is the main function of the iliotibial tract.

 d. False As its name implies, the iliotibial tract inserts into the lateral condyle of the tibia.

 e. True The superior gluteal nerve supplies gluteus medius, minimus and tensor fascia lata.

12. The gluteal region:
a. Comprises the three gluteal muscles, piriformis, obturator externus, the two gemelli and quadratus femoris.
b. Is delineated by the fold of the buttock which corresponds to the lower border of gluteus maximus.
c. Includes the gluteus maximus muscle which has some fibres inserting into the gluteal crest of the femur.
d. Includes the gluteus maximus which is the largest of the three gluteal muscles and is therefore supplied by both the superior and inferior gluteal nerves.
e. Includes gluteus medius and minimus, both of which arise from the gluteal surface of the ilium.

13. The femoral triangle:
a. Is bounded by the inguinal ligament, the medial border of sartorius and the lateral border of adductor longus.
b. Contains the femoral vessels and nerve.
c. Contains iliacus, psoas and quadratus femoris in its floor.
d. Contains a branch of the femoral nerve which supplies the pectineus muscle.
e. Contains the femoral artery from which the medial and lateral circumflex femoral arteries arise.

14. Piriformis:
a. Arises from all five sacral segments.
b. Emerges through the lesser sciatic foramen to insert into the greater trochanter of the femur.
c. Is supplied by the ventral rami of $S_{1,2}$.
d. Plays a role in stabilizing the hip joint, especially in abduction.
e. Has the sacral plexus lying on its dorsal surface.

12. a. False The muscles of the gluteal region are the three gluteal muscles, piriformis, obturator *internus*, the two gemelli and quadratus femoris.

    b. False The gluteal fold is the posterior horizontal skin crease indicating the level of the hip joint.

    c. True The rest of its fibres insert into the iliotibial tract.

    d. False Gluteus maximus is the largest of the three gluteal muscles, but it is supplied only by the inferior gluteal nerve.

    e. True All the gluteal muscles arise from the gluteal surface of the ilium.

13. a. False The femoral triangle is bounded by the inguinal ligament above, the medial border of sartorius laterally, and the *medial* border of adductor longus medially.

    b. True The nerve divides into its terminal branches in this region, and the vessels pass into the adductor canal.

    c. False It is iliacus, psoas and *pectineus* which lie in the floor of the femoral triangle, in addition to a narrow strip of adductor brevis.

    d. True Pectineus usually has an additional nerve supply from the obturator nerve.

    e. False The medial and lateral circumflex femoral arteries arise from the profunda femoris artery.

14. a. False It arises from the middle three sacral segments.

    b. False It emerges from the *greater* sciatic foramen to insert into the greater trochanter of the femur.

    c. True It is supplied segmentally by small branches from the upper two sacral nerves.

    d. True This is the role of all the short muscles acting on the hip joint. Piriformis itself is a lateral rotator of the joint.

    e. False The sacral plexus lies on the *ventral* surface of piriformis.

15. The capsule of the hip joint:
  a. Is strengthened by three ligaments, one arising from each of the three bones which make up the pelvis.
  b. Is strengthened by the ischiofemoral ligament, which is the strongest of the three and prevents posterior dislocation of the hip.
  c. Is attached circumferentially to the acetabular labrum and the transverse ligament, which closes the acetabular notch.
  d. Is attached to the femur at the intertrochanteric line anteriorly and the intertrochanteric crest posteriorly.
  e. Contains the ligamentum teres (ligament of the head of the femur) which is attached to the iliopubic eminence in the centre of the acetabulum.

16. The hip joint:
  a. Receives a large proportion of its blood supply from the artery in the ligament of the head of the femur.
  b. Is innervated by each of the three major nerves that supply the lower limb.
  c. Receives a branch of the femoral nerve via the nerve to quadratus femoris.
  d. Receives blood via the trochanteric anastomosis which is derived from both gluteal and both circumflex femoral arteries.
  e. Is a site of direct contact between the femoral vessels and the capsule of the joint anteriorly.

17. The ligaments of the knee joint:
  a. Include the fibular collateral ligament which is attached to the lateral epicondyle of the femur, the lateral meniscus and the head of the fibula.
  b. Include the tibial collateral ligament which is made up of a superficial and deep part, the latter being a thickening of the capsule of the knee joint.
  c. Include the posterior cruciate ligament which is of great importance in walking downhill or downstairs.
  d. Receive their blood supply mainly through the genicular branches of the popliteal artery.
  e. Include the anterior and posterior cruciate ligaments which lie within the synovial cavity of the knee joint.

15. a. True They are the iliofemoral, pubofemoral and ischiofemoral ligaments.

b. False The ischiofemoral ligament is the weakest of the three. It is the iliofemoral ligament (the Y-shaped ligament of Bigelow) which is the strongest.

c. True This is the site of attachment of the capsule of the hip joint to the pelvis.

d. False The capsule attaches to the intertrochanteric line anteriorly, but only extends halfway down the neck of the femur posteriorly.

e. False The ligamentum teres attaches to the transverse ligament, which closes the acetabular notch.

16. a. False The artery in the ligamentum teres provides an insignificant volume of blood to the head of the femur and the hip joint.

b. True Hilton's law states that the nerve which supplies a muscle will also give a branch to the joint which is moved by that muscle (and another branch to the skin overlying it).

c. False Quadratus femoris is supplied by the sciatic nerve which provides a twig supplying the hip joint.

d. True This is the main source of blood for the head of the femur and the capsule of the hip joint.

e. False The capsule of the hip joint is separated anteriorly from the femoral vessels by the iliacus muscle and the tendon of the psoas major muscle.

17. a. False The fibular collateral ligament is not attached to the lateral meniscus. This is thought to be one of the reasons why the lateral meniscus is injured less often than the medial meniscus.

b. True It is this deep portion which is attached firmly to the medial meniscus and restricts its mobility.

c. True The posterior cruciate ligament prevents the femur from slipping forwards when the knee is flexed and weight-bearing.

d. True The popliteal artery usually has five genicular branches. They are the medial and lateral superior genicular arteries, the middle genicular artery and the medial and lateral inferior genicular arteries.

e. False The cruciate ligaments are intracapsular but extrasynovial.

18. **The extensor compartment of the leg:**
    a. Includes tibialis anterior which arises from the lateral aspect of the upper fibula.
    b. Includes extensor hallucis longus, which is innervated by $L_{4,5}$.
    c. Includes peroneus longus and brevis which evert the foot.
    d. Includes tibialis anterior whose tendon is a prominent landmark on the medial aspect of the dorsum of the foot.
    e. Includes peroneus tertius which is absent in a number of normal individuals.

19. **The deep peroneal nerve:**
    a. Supplies all the muscles of the extensor compartment of the leg.
    b. Supplies all the muscles of the lateral compartment of the leg.
    c. Carries motor fibres only.
    d. Passes over the neck of the fibula, where it can be damaged in fractures at this site.
    e. Lies in close proximity to the posterior tibial artery throughout its course.

18. a. False It arises from the upper tibia and the interosseous membrane.

    b. True It is of paramount importance to test the power of extensor hallucis longus (by asking the patient to dorsiflex the big toe against resistance) in cases of suspected lumbar disc prolapse, as this is one of the earliest signs of compression of the relevant lumbar nerve root.

    c. False These two peronei are not extensors of the foot and therefore are not part of the extensor compartment. They lie in the lateral compartment of the leg.

    d. True The other prominent tendon on the dorsum of the foot is the tendon of extensor digitorum longus which lies lateral to it.

    e. True Peroneus tertius is an extensor of the foot and does lie in the extensor compartment. It arises as a lateral slip from extensor digitorum longus and inserts on to the fifth metatarsal.

19. a. True The muscles of the extensor compartment are tibialis anterior, extensor hallucis longus, extensor digitorum longus and peroneus tertius, and they are all supplied by the deep peroneal nerve.

    b. False The muscles of the lateral compartment are peroneus longus and brevis and they are both supplied by the *superficial* peroneal nerve.

    c. False It carries sensation from the periosteum of the lower tibia and fibula and the skin on the dorsum of the foot between the big and index toes.

    d. True The nerve can also be damaged by a tight plaster cast in this region.

    e. False It closely follows the course of the *anterior* tibial artery.

20. The lateral compartment of the leg:

a. Contains the peroneus longus muscle which everts and weakly dorsiflexes the foot.
b. Contains peroneus brevis which arises from both the tibia and the fibula.
c. Contains tibialis posterior which plantar flexes the foot.
d. Contains peroneus longus and brevis whose tendons are bound down by the superior and inferior peroneal retinacula.
e. Contains peroneus longus and brevis which are both supplied by the superficial peroneal nerve which has a root value of L_5S_1.

21. The posterior compartment of the leg:

a. Receives sensory supply of its overlying skin from the posterior femoral cutaneous nerve exclusively.
b. Includes plantaris which is one of the main flexors of the ankle joint.
c. Comprises three muscles lying superficially which have a common insertion on the posterior surface of the calcaneum.
d. Includes in the deep group flexor hallucis longus and flexor digitorum longus, both of which are supplied by branches from the tibial nerve ($S_{1,2}$), and tibialis posterior, which also receives its nerve supply from the tibial nerve (L_4).
e. Includes gastrocnemius which lies deep to soleus.

20. a. False Peroneus longus inserts into the base of the
metatarsal of the big toe on the plantar surface of
the foot. It therefore everts and plantar flexes the
foot.

b. False Peroneus brevis arises from the lower fibula only
and does not take origin from the tibia.

c. False Tibialis posterior does plantar flex the foot. It lies,
however, in the posterior compartment of the leg.

d. True These retinacula prevent the peroneal tendons from
slipping from their positions behind the lateral
malleolus and below the peroneal trochlea
respectively.

e. True The power of eversion and inversion must also be
checked in the clinical assessment of a suspected
prolapsed lumbosacral disc.

21. a. False The skin of the calf is supplied by the posterior
femoral cutaneous nerve in its upper half, the sural
nerve supplies the lower half, the saphenous nerve
supplies the medial aspect and communicating
branches from the common peroneal nerve supply
the lateral aspect.

b. False Plantaris is a vestigial muscle, i.e. a muscle which is
disappearing in the human race. It has a very small
belly and a long thin tendon, and its contraction
would contribute only marginally towards flexing
the ankle joint. It is homologous to palmaris longus
in the forearm.

c. True The three muscles of the superficial group are
gastrocnemius, soleus and plantaris and they all
insert via the tendo calcaneus (Achilles tendon) into
the posterior surface of the calcaneum.

d. True Tibialis posterior is an inverter of the foot and is
supplied by the L_4 spinal cord segment. The long
flexors of the toes however receive their innervation
from the upper two sacral spinal cord segments,
even though the nerve fibres reach them all via the
same nerve – the tibial, which has the root value
$L_{4,5}S_{1-3}$.

e. False Gastrocnemius lies superficial to soleus.

22. In the sole of the foot:
    a.   The muscles lie deep to the plantar aponeurosis which arises from the calcaneum and is inserted into the proximal phalanx of each of the five toes.
    b.   The muscles in the first layer are the flexors of the toes, including the flexors of the big and little toe.
    c.   Abductor digiti minimi and flexor digitorum brevis are supplied by the lateral plantar nerve.
    d.   The second layer of muscles contains the tendons of the long flexors of the toes and the big toe.
    e.   Flexor accessorius (quadratus plantae) arises by two heads from the calcaneum.

23. In the sole of the foot:
    a.   The lumbricals, which arise from the tendons of flexor digitorum brevis, lie in the second layer of muscles.
    b.   Both flexor digiti minimi brevis and longus are innervated by the lateral plantar nerve.
    c.   Adductor hallucis has a transverse and oblique head.
    d.   The deepest layer contains only the interossei.
    e.   The tendon of tibialis posterior is inserted into the base of the talus.

24. The blood supply of the sole of the foot:
    a.   Is via the medial and lateral plantar arteries which are the terminal branches of the anterior tibial artery.
    b.   Is via the superficial and deep plantar arches.
    c.   Is derived from the arteries which lie between the first and second layers of the sole of the foot.
    d.   Reaches the toes via digital arteries which arise mainly from the medial plantar artery.
    e.   Receives a contribution from the dorsalis pedis artery.

22. a. True The plantar aponeurosis is similar in consistency and function to the palmar aponeurosis in the hand.

b. False The muscles of the first layer are the short flexor of the toes (flexor digitorum brevis) and the abductors of the big and little toes. The short flexors of the big and little toes lie in the third layer.

c. False Abductor digiti minimi is supplied by the lateral plantar nerve. Flexor digitorum brevis, however, is supplied by the medial plantar nerve.

d. True The tendons of flexor digitorum longus and flexor hallucis longus lie in the second layer.

e. True The medial head is fleshy and the lateral head is tendinous.

23. a. False The lumbricals do lie in the second layer. However, they arise from the tendons of flexor digitorum longus.

b. False Flexor digiti minimi longus is a muscle which does not exist! Flexor digiti minimi brevis is only called brevis to differentiate it from flexor digiti minimi, which is in the hand!

c. True They both adduct the big toe.

d. False It contains the interossei and the tendons of tibialis posterior and peroneus longus.

e. False The tendon of the tibialis posterior inserts into the tuberosity of the navicular which lies on the medial aspect of the foot.

24. a. False The medial and lateral plantar arteries are the terminal branches of the posterior tibial artery.

b. False There is only one arterial arch in the sole of the foot and it is called the plantar arch.

c. True The neurovascular plane of the sole of the foot lies between the first and second layer, superficial to the long flexor tendons of the toes.

d. False It is the lateral plantar artery which is the larger of the two. It gives rise to the plantar arch from which most of the digital arteries arise. The blood in the medial plantar artery is destined mainly for the big toe.

e. True This is via perforating branches of the arcuate artery which contribute to the plantar arch.

25. At the ankle joint:
  a. Dorsiflexion, plantar flexion, inversion and eversion are the possible movements.
  b. The deltoid ligament extends from the medial malleolus of the tibia to the medial cuneiform.
  c. There are three ligaments connecting the lateral malleolus of the fibula to the talus and the calcaneus.
  d. The blood supply is via the anterior and posterior tibial arteries and the peroneal artery.
  e. It is a synovial joint between the lower ends of the tibia and fibula, and the articular surfaces of the talus and navicular bones.

26. The hip bone:
  a. Is made up of three bones which all come together in the acetabulum.
  b. Articulates with the sacrum posteriorly in a secondary cartilaginous joint which permits very little movement.
  c. Receives the insertion of psoas major which arises from the lumbar vertebrae.
  d. Gives origin to rectus femoris which arises by two heads from the anterior superior iliac spine and the superior pubic ramus.
  e. Has the anterior superior iliac spine and the pubic tubercle in the same vertical plane in the anatomical position.

25. a. False Inversion and eversion occur at the mid tarsal and subtalar joints.
  b. False The deltoid ligament has a deep part which extends from the medial malleolus to the talus, and a superficial part which extends from the medial malleolus to the talus, sustentaculum tali of the calcaneus and the navicular bone.
  c. True They are the anterior and posterior talofibular ligaments and the calcaneofibular ligament which lies between the two.
  d. True The ankle joint receives its blood supply from all the arteries in the region.
  e. False The navicular bone does not take part in the ankle joint.

26. a. True The ilium, pubis and ischium all contribute to the acetabulum.
  b. False The sacroiliac joint permits very little movement, but it is a synovial joint which can often become fibrous in adults.
  c. False Psoas major inserts into the lesser trochanter of the femur.
  d. False The rectus femoris arises from the anterior inferior iliac spine and the ilium above the acetabulum.
  e. True This is the position in which the dry bone should be held during viva exams!

27. The hip bone:
a.   Has a greater and lesser sciatic notch which transmit the superior and inferior gluteal nerves respectively.
b.   Has the iliac crest whose highest point reaches the level of the second lumbar vertebra.
c.   Joins the hip bone of the other side by means of a synovial joint between the two pubic bones.
d.   Contains numerous strong fibrous bands within the cavity of the sacroiliac joint which connect the two articular surfaces.
e.   Carries the ischial spine which separates the greater and lesser sciatic notches.

28. The pubis:
a.   Has an inferior ramus which joins the ilium and ischium to form the acetabulum.
b.   Has an inferior ramus which forms the medial and lateral borders of the obturator foramen.
c.   Has the pubic crest on the upper part of its body which gives rise to the rectus abdominis.
d.   Gives origin to all the adductors of the lower limb except part of adductor magnus.
e.   Has the pubic tubercle which receives the attachment of the inguinal ligament.

27. a. False   The notches are transformed into foramina by the sacrotuberous and sacrospinous ligaments. The superior and inferior gluteal nerves both pass with piriformis through the greater sciatic foramen.

    b. False   The highest point of the iliac crest is a very important anatomical landmark as it lies at the level of the disc between L_4 and L_5 vertebrae, a level which is considered safe for performing lumbar punctures.

    c. False   The two pubic bones are joined at the symphysis pubis, which is a secondary cartilaginous joint.

    d. True   They produce the pitting which can be seen clearly on the articular surfaces of both the sacrum and the ilium.

    e. True   This is another important anatomical landmark which can be palpated during vaginal examination. Its clinical importance is that it lies just above the pudendal nerve and therefore in pudendal nerve blocks, e.g. prior to episiotomy, the needle delivering the local anaesthetic should be directed towards the ischial spine.

28. a. False   It is the *superior* pubic ramus which contributes to the acetabulum.

    b. False   The inferior ramus of the pubis forms the medial border of the obturator foramen; the lateral border is formed by the inferior ramus of the ischium.

    c. True   The linea alba is attached to the symphysis pubis which lies between the two pubic crests.

    d. True   Gracilis, adductors longus, brevis and part of magnus all arise from the pubis. The hamstring portion of adductor magnus arises from the ischium.

    e. True   Of utmost importance in hernia repairs.

29. The femur:
  a. Has two trochanters, each of which ossifies as a separate epiphysis.
  b. Has a greater trochanter which provides attachment to piriformis.
  c. Has the lesser trochanter which provides attachment to gluteus maximus.
  d. Has on the anterior surface of the shaft the linea aspera which provides attachment for adductor magnus.
  e. Has a popliteal surface which lies between the two supracondylar lines and provides origin for the popliteus muscle.

30. The lower end of the femur:
  a. Has a medial condyle which projects further forwards than the lateral, thus preventing medial dislocation of the patella.
  b. Has the attachment of the anterior cruciate ligament posteriorly on the inner surface of the lateral condyle.
  c. Has the attachment of the posterior cruciate ligament anteriorly on the inner surface of the lateral condyle of the femur.
  d. Has plantaris which arises from the upper part of the lateral condyle.
  e. Has the adductor tubercle on its medial aspect.

29. a. True Both centres of ossification appear during childhood.
  b. True Piriformis extends from the middle three sacral segments to the greater trochanter of the femur.
  c. False The lesser trochanter provides attachment to the psoas tendon. Gluteus maximus is inserted into the gluteal tuberosity and the iliotibial tract.
  d. False The linea aspera does provide attachment for adductor magnus; however, it lies on the *posterior* surface of the shaft of the femur.
  e. False The popliteal surface is bare. The popliteus muscle arises from the popliteal surface of the tibia and inserts into the lateral meniscus of the knee joint and the lateral condyle of the femur.

30. a. False It is the lateral condyle of the femur which extends further forwards. The patella tends to become dislocated laterally, and all the preventive mechanisms are geared towards preventing its *lateral* dislocation. The lowest fibres of vastus medialis are almost horizontal to achieve that aim.
  b. True The anterior and posterior cruciate ligaments are named according to their site of origin on the tibial plateau. As they cross each other (in a cruciate manner), the anterior cruciate eventually inserts posteriorly on the inner surface of the lateral condyle of the femur.
  c. False The posterior cruciate ligament inserts anteriorly on the inner surface of the *medial* condyle of the femur.
  d. True The lateral head of gastrocnemius and the fibular collateral ligament also arise from the lateral condyle below the origin of plantaris.
  e. True It provides insertion for the hamstring fibres of adductor magnus.

31. The patella:
    a. Is the largest sesamoid bone in the body.
    b. Has a smooth outer surface.
    c. Ossifies from one centre only, which appears in the seventh year.
    d. Overlies the knee joint which is at the level of the middle of the patella.
    e. Is attached distally to the tuberosity of the tibia by means of the patellar ligament.

32. The tibia:
    a. Articulates with the fibula at the tibial plateau.
    b. Has the medial and lateral menisci lying on its superior articular surface separated by the tibial spine.
    c. Has the muscles of the extensor compartment of the leg lying anterior to the interosseous membrane.
    d. Has tibialis anterior arising from its subcutaneous surface.
    e. Has the soleal line on its posterior surface which gives origin to the fibres of soleus and gastrocnemius.

31. a. True It is classified as a sesamoid bone as it lies in the quadriceps tendon.

   b. True The inner surface is identified by the medial and lateral articular surfaces.

   c. False Ossification is usually from one centre only, but may be from two or three centres, leading to a bi- or tripartite patella which can be misinterpreted as a fracture on X-ray. The ossification centre appears at about 3 years of age.

   d. False The lower border of the patella overlies the knee joint.

   e. True It is this tendon which is tapped when eliciting the knee-jerk reflex.

32. a. False The tibial plateau (superior articular surface) articulates with the menisci and the condyles of the femur.

   b. True The anterior and posterior cruciate ligaments arise anterior and posterior to this spine respectively.

   c. True The interosseous membrane extends from the medial aspect of the tibia to the fibula and the muscles of the extensor compartment lie anterior to it.

   d. False The subcutaneous surface is subcutaneous and has no muscles arising from it.

   e. False The soleal line gives origin to soleus (which also takes origin from the fibula). Gastrocnemius, however, arises via its medial and lateral heads from the lower end of the femur.

33. The fibula:
   a. Articulates with the tibia by means of a synovial joint superiorly and a fibrous joint inferiorly.
   b. Has a styloid process on its head which provides attachment for the fibular collateral ligament.
   c. Has the lateral malleolus at its lower end which articulates with the talus and calcaneum.
   d. Has the tendons of peroneus brevis, longus and tertius passing behind its lateral malleolus.
   e. Gives origin to both flexor and extensor hallucis longus.

34. The tarsus:
   a. Like the carpus, is made up of eight bones.
   b. Has all its bones, except the talus, resting on the ground to provide weight-bearing.
   c. Includes the talus, which has the sustentaculum tali as a prominent feature.
   d. Includes the calcaneus, which articulates with the cuboid.
   e. Includes the talus, which has articular surfaces for the tibia and fibula, the calcaneus, navicular and cuboid bones.

35. The following tendons are associated with sesamoid bones:
   a. Quadriceps femoris.
   b. Lateral head of gastrocnemius.
   c. Flexor hallucis longus.
   d. Peroneus longus.
   e. Tibialis posterior.

33. a. True The superior tibiofibular joint is a synovial joint and the inferior tibiofibular joint is a fibrous joint. The latter is sometimes classed as the only true syndesmosis in the body.

 b. False The fibular collateral ligament is attached to the head of the fibula. It is the arcuate popliteal ligament which is attached to the styloid process.

 c. False The tibia and fibula articulate with the talus to form the ankle joint. The calcaneum is not part of this joint.

 d. False The tendon of peroneus tertius does not pass behind the lateral malleolus. It is considered as part of the extensor compartment of the leg.

 e. True Extensor hallucis longus arises from its extensor surface and flexor hallucis longus arises from its flexor surface.

34. a. False There are only seven bones in the tarsus – the calcaneus, talus, navicular, cuboid and three cuneiforms.

 b. False The calcaneus is the only tarsal bone which rests on the ground.

 c. False The sustentaculum tali is part of the calcaneus. It is the support of the talus.

 d. True This is at the calcaneocuboid joint, which is part of the mid tarsal joint.

 e. False The talus does not articulate with the cuboid.

35. a. True It carries the patella, the largest sesamoid bone in the body.

 b. False There is a sesamoid bone, the fabella, often present in the lateral head of gastrocnemius, which is a muscle, not a tendon.

 c. False It is flexor hallucis *brevis* which is typically associated with not one, but two sesamoid bones.

 d. True It is usually present in the groove on the inferior surface of the cuboid.

 e. True It is usually present at the level of the head of the talus.

36. The talus:
a. Articulates with the navicular at the talonavicular joint and with the calcaneus at a separate joint – the talocalcaneal joint.
b. Has the sustentaculum tali supporting it on its inferolateral aspect.
c. Has both parts of the deltoid ligament attached to its medial surface.
d. Does not attach to the spring ligament.
e. Has an extensive blood supply from both the anterior and posterior tibial arteries and therefore very rarely undergoes avascular necrosis after dislocation.

37. The inguinal lymph nodes receive lymph from:
a. The big toe.
b. The buttock.
c. The anterior abdominal wall.
d. The scrotum.
e. The testes.

38. A patient was stabbed in the inguinal region and sustained a complete section of his femoral nerve. On examination several weeks after the injury, he was found to have:
a. Inability to extend the knee.
b. Wasting of the anterior compartment of the thigh.
c. An abnormal gait.
d. Altered sensation below the knee.
e. Asymmetrical buttocks.

36. a. False The talocalcaneonavicular joint is one joint with a single synovial cavity which has two components – the talonavicular and talocalcaneal parts.

   b. False The sustentaculum tali is part of the calcaneus and lies underneath the talus below the medial malleolus.

   c. True Both the deep and superficial parts of the deltoid ligament are attached to the medial aspect of the talus.

   d. False The spring ligament attaches to the talus at the talocalcaneonavicular joint.

   e. False The talus does have numerous vascular foramina and does receive its blood supply from both tibial arteries. However, these blood vessels are usually ruptured when the talus is dislocated and therefore avascular necrosis of the talus is very common after dislocation.

37. a. True The lymphatic drainage of the inguinal lymph nodes can be remembered by means of the mnemonic: before, below, behind, between. The entire lower limb is the 'below'.

   b. True This is the 'behind'.

   c. True This is the 'before'.

   d. True This is included in the 'between'.

   e. False The testes drain back to the para-aortic lymph nodes at the level of the origin of the testicular arteries.

38. a. True The femoral nerve supplies the quadriceps femoris which extends the knee joint.

   b. True The muscles of the anterior compartment would have atrophied if their nerve supply had been cut a few weeks before examination.

   c. True The patient would be able to walk by tilting his pelvis, but his gait would certainly be very unusual.

   d. True The saphenous nerve, which is the terminal branch of the femoral nerve, is sensory to the skin of the medial aspect of the foot and the leg below the knee.

   e. False The gluteal muscles are supplied by the superior and inferior gluteal nerves and would be unaffected in an injury involving the femoral nerve.

39. Inversion of the foot:
 a. Is equivalent to supination in the upper limb.
 b. Enables human beings to walk up and downhill.
 c. Is performed mainly by tibialis anterior and posterior.
 d. Is opposed by the three peronei.
 e. Occurs at the mid tarsal and subtalar joints.

40. The bursae around the knee joint:
 a. Are four in number anteriorly.
 b. Are four in number laterally.
 c. Include a bursa beneath the semimembranosus tendon which forms a fluctuating swelling behind the knee which can disappear during extension.
 d. Include the suprapatellar bursa which develops as several bursae in the fetus which coalesce.
 e. Include the deep infrapatellar bursa which is involved in housemaid's knee.

39. a. True   Due to adaptation of the human lower limb for weight-bearing, supination of the lower limb is not as full as in the upper limb.

    b. False It is the movements of the knee and ankle joint which are mainly responsible for walking up and downhill. The ability to invert and evert the foot enables human beings to walk on uneven surfaces.

    c. True   They are assisted by flexor and extensor hallucis longus.

    d. True   Peroneus longus, brevis and tertius are evertors of the foot and therefore oppose inversion.

    e. True   Inversion and eversion begin in the mid tarsal joint. When all possible movement in that joint has taken place, any further movement which occurs will be at the subtalar joints.

40. a. True   They are the subcutaneous prepatellar, the deep infrapatellar, the subcutaneous infrapatellar and the suprapatellar.

    b. True   They are the bursa between the lateral head of gastrocnemius and the capsule of the knee joint, the bursa between the fibular collateral ligament and the tendon of biceps femoris, the bursa between the same ligament and the tendon of popliteus and the bursa between the same tendon and the lateral condyle of the femur.

    c. False It disappears during *flexion* of the knee joint and often communicates with its synovial cavity.

    d. False It forms as a single bursa. It often communicates with the synovial cavity of the knee joint.

    e. False It is the prepatellar bursa which is involved in housemaid's knee. The infrapatellar bursae are involved when kneeling in a more erect posture (clergyman's knee).

Thorax

1. **Blood supplying the heart:**
    a. Passes via the right and left coronary arteries which arise from the right and left aortic sinuses respectively.
    b. Passes via the anterior interventricular artery which arises from the right coronary artery.
    c. All drains into the coronary sinus.
    d. After its passage through the myocardium, blood in the coronary sinus passes to the right atrium in close proximity to the opening of the superior vena cava.
    e. Includes potential anastomoses between coronary arteries and pericardial arteries.

2. **The breast:**
    a. Is a modified apocrine sebaceous gland.
    b. In the female has a base which extends from the second to the sixth rib in the mid clavicular line.
    c. Has about six to eight main ducts which open through a common orifice on the summit of the nipple.
    d. Receives its blood supply mainly from the internal thoracic artery.
    e. Has a lymph drainage to the axillary and infraclavicular lymph nodes from its lateral part, and to the internal thoracic lymph nodes from its medial part.

3. **The thoracic muscles:**
    a. Include the external intercostal muscles which run downwards and backwards.
    b. Include the serratus posterior superior and serratus posterior inferior which are part of the intermediate layer.
    c. Include the transversus (innermost) layer which is made up of three groups of muscles.
    d. Are supplied by the intercostal vessels which run between the external and intermediate layers.
    e. Include the innermost intercostals which cross more than one intercostal space.

1. a. False They arise from the anterior and left posterior
               aortic sinuses.
    b. False It arises from the left coronary artery. The right
               coronary artery gives rise to the posterior
               interventricular artery and the circumflex branch.
    c. False The anterior cardiac veins open directly into the
               right atrium.
    d. False The coronary sinus opens into the right atrium in
               close proximity to the opening of the inferior vena
               cava.
    e. True   The pericardial arteries, which are derived from
               pericardiacophrenic, bronchial and internal thoracic
               arteries, may in rare instances open up to replace a
               coronary artery. Effectively, coronary arteries are
               end-arteries.

2. a. False It is a modified apocrine *sweat* gland.
    b. True   The size of the *base* of the breast is fairly constant
               in most individuals.
    c. False There are usually about 15 main ducts, and they
               open separately on the summit of the nipple.
    d. False The blood supply of the breast is mainly from the
               lateral thoracic artery from the axillary artery.
    e. True   This is the basic principle of lymph drainage of the
               breast, but other pathways are possible, especially
               in the event of obstruction due to malignancy.
               Lymph drainage may then pass to the opposite
               breast, cervical lymph nodes, peritoneal cavity and
               even the inguinal lymph nodes.

3. a. False They run downwards and *forwards* in a similar
               direction to the fibres of the external oblique (see
               Abdomen question 2).
    b. False These two muscles, along with the external
               intercostals, make up the outer thoracic layer of
               muscles.
    c. True   They are the subcostal, the innermost intercostal
               and the transversus thoracis muscles.
    d. False The neurovascular plane lies between the
               intermediate and innermost layers.
    e. True   This applies to all the muscles in the innermost
               layer.

4. **The diaphragm:**
   a. Receives its blood supply from the lowest two intercostal arteries.
   b. Has the greater, lesser and least splanchnic nerves passing behind the median arcuate ligament.
   c. Has the subcostal vessels and nerve passing behind the lateral arcuate ligament.
   d. Contracts in inspiration and relaxes in expiration.
   e. Has the opening of the inferior vena cava in its central tendon.

5. **The mediastinum:**
   a. Includes the superior mediastinum, which lies above the thoracic inlet.
   b. Includes the inferior mediastinum, which is divided into the anterior and posterior mediastinum.
   c. Includes the superior mediastinum, which has the oesophagus lying against the body of C_6.
   d. Contains the arch of the aorta, which extends from the anterior mediastinum, rises into the superior mediastinum and then descends into the posterior mediastinum.
   e. Contains the right and left brachiocephalic veins, which lie superficial to the arteries.

6. **At the level of T_4:**
   a. The trachea bifurcates into the right and left main bronchi.
   b. The azygos vein enters the inferior vena cava.
   c. The thoracic duct lies to the right of the oesophagus.
   d. The second costal cartilage articulates with the sternum.
   e. The ligamentum arteriosum connects the arch of the aorta to the pulmonary trunk.

4. a. False It is supplied by the lower five intercostal arteries, the subcostal and musculophrenic arteries, and the right and left inferior phrenic arteries.
    b. False They pass behind the crura of the diaphragm on their respective sides.
    c. True   They can be seen on the posterior abdominal wall emerging from behind the diaphragm laterally.
    d. True   The upwards movement of the diaphragm in expiration is due to pressure of the abdominal contents.
    e. True   The wall of the inferior vena cava is firmly attached to the caval opening in the central tendon of the diaphragm.

5. a. False The superior mediastinum lies between the thoracic inlet and a horizontal plane lying at the level of the sternal angle.
    b. False It is divided into anterior, middle and posterior mediastinum.
    c. False By definition, the thoracic inlet starts at the level of T_1.
    d. False The arch of the aorta lies entirely in the superior mediastinum.
    e. True   This follows the general principle that veins run superficial to the arteries.

6. a. True   This is the level of the bifurcation of the trachea, behind the sternal angle.
    b. False The azygos vein enters the *superior* vena cava at this level.
    c. False At this level, the thoracic duct has passed behind, and reached the left side of the oesophagus.
    d. True   The sternal angle lies at the level of the lower border of the fourth thoracic vertebra.
    e. False It connects the left pulmonary artery to the aortic arch.

7. **The trachea:**
   a. Commences in the neck at the level of C_4.
   b. Extends from the lower end of the cricoid cartilage to the level of the sternal angle.
   c. Has a thoracic portion which lies in the anterior mediastinum.
   d. Receives its nerve supply from both vagi and recurrent laryngeal nerves in addition to sympathetic fibres.
   e. Receives its blood supply via numerous small branches arising directly from both external carotid arteries segmentally.

8. **The thymus:**
   a. Is the principal content of the anterior mediastinum.
   b. Overlies the commencement of the superior vena cava.
   c. Derives its blood supply from the thymic artery, which is a sizeable vessel in children.
   d. Drains lymph from the mediastinal lymph nodes.
   e. Regresses in early infancy and is replaced by fibrous tissue.

9. **The diaphragm:**
   a. Transmits the aorta at the level of the 10th thoracic vertebra.
   b. Receives its motor supply from the phrenic nerves, which have a root value of C_{2-4}.
   c. Has a left crus which encircles the oesophageal opening and contributes to the lower oesophageal sphincter.
   d. Takes origin from the medial and lateral arcuate ligaments, which are the thickened upper margin of the fascia covering psoas major and quadratus lumborum respectively.
   e. Receives a sensory supply from the lower five intercostal nerves.

7. a. False It commences at the level of C_6.
    b. True These are the surface markings of the trachea.
    c. False The thoracic trachea lies in the superior mediastinum. It bifurcates before reaching the posterior mediastinum.
    d. True The vagi provide parasympathetic innervation and supply the mucous membrane of the trachea.
    e. False It is supplied by branches from the inferior thyroid and bronchial arteries.

8. a. True It may, however, lie in the anterior part of the superior mediastinum and extend up into the neck. The other components of the anterior mediastinum are the sternopericardial ligaments.
    b. True This is in the superior mediastinum, at the level of the junction of the first costal cartilage and the manubrium sterni on the right side.
    c. False The thymus is certainly larger in children; however, its blood supply is from the inferior thyroid and internal thoracic arteries.
    d. False The thymus receives no afferent lymphatics.
    e. False It regresses after puberty and is replaced by fatty tissue; however, it does not necessarily disappear completely.

9. a. False The aorta passes through the diaphragm at the level of the 12th thoracic vertebra. The oesophagus pierces it at T_{10}, and the inferior vena cava at T_8.
    b. False The root value of the phrenic nerve is C_{3-5}. The mnemonic is $C_{3,4 \text{ and } 5}$, keeps my diaphragm alive (see Pelvis question 21 for the second part of the mnemonic).
    c. False It is the right crus which encircles the oesophageal opening. It is also the larger of the two crura, as it arises from the bodies of L_{1-3}, whereas the left crus arises from the bodies of $L_{1,2}$ only.
    d. True It also arises from the lower part of the sternum, the lower six ribs and their costal cartilages and the first three lumbar vertebrae via the crura.
    e. True The lower five intercostal nerves supply the periphery of the diaphragm, whereas the central part receives its sensory supply from the phrenic nerves.

10. The ribs:
   a. Articulate with costal cartilages that make synovial joints with the sternum.
   b. Articulate with costal cartilages in secondary cartilaginous joints.
   c. Are involved in rotation of their necks at all 12 costovertebral joints.
   d. Are connected to the transverse processes of the vertebrae above by means of the costotransverse ligaments.
   e. Have heads to which are attached three ligaments.

11. In the typical intercostal space:
   a. There is a collateral branch of the intercostal nerve which is purely sensory.
   b. The main nerve passes between the innermost and internal intercostal muscles.
   c. Some of the arterial supply arises from the internal thoracic artery.
   d. Some venous drainage is via the posterior intercostal veins into the azygous system.
   e. Lymphatic drainage of the posterior part of the space is to posterior intercostal nodes.

10. a. False The first chondrosternal joint is primary
cartilaginous, whilst the rest are synovial. The next
six articulate separately, and the eighth, ninth and
10th articulate with the sternum via a single
synovial joint.

b. False The joints formed between the costal cartilages and
their ribs are primary cartilaginous joints.

c. True Such rotation results in elevation or depression of
the anterior ends of the respective ribs.

d. False Only the superior (and not the inferior or lateral)
costotransverse ligament is attached to the vertebra
above; the latter two are attached to the vertebra at
the same level.

e. True These are the so-called triradiate ligaments.

11. a. False The collateral nerve is solely motor.

b. True This can only be true, however, where there is an
innermost intercostal muscle, i.e. only in the lateral
wall of the thorax.

c. True Some arterial blood reaches the intercostal spaces
via the anterior intercostal arteries from the internal
thoracic artery. The posterior parts of the spaces are
supplied by the posterior intercostal arteries, being
direct branches of the thoracic aorta. The posterior
parts of the first two spaces, however, are supplied
by blood derived from the costocervical trunk,
a branch of the second part of the subclavian artery.

d. True The first space is drained by the supreme intercostal
vein into the vertebral vein or brachiocephalic vein.
The drainage of the second (and third) spaces is
via the superior intercostal veins via the azygos
vein on the right and the brachiocephalic vein on
the left side. The rest drain via the azygos,
hemiazygos or accessory hemiazygos veins.

e. True They lie alongside the thoracic aorta.

12. The diaphragm:
    a.   Is supplied by the lower nine intercostal arteries in its costal margin.
    b.   Has its caval opening opposite the eighth thoracic vertebra.
    c.   Has the sympathetic trunk passing posterior to the crus.
    d.   Has its central tendon level with the third right costal cartilage.
    e.   Transmits the thoracic duct via the aortic opening.

13. In the superior mediastinum:
    a.   The oesophagus lies against the body of the first thoracic vertebra.
    b.   The arch of the aorta lies partly in the superior and partly in the inferior mediastinum.
    c.   The superior vena cava passes inferiorly, posterior to the left border of the sternum.
    d.   The dead space is mainly on the left.
    e.   The superior vena cava receives the azygos vein opposite the fifth right costal cartilage.

12. a. False The costal margin of the diaphragm is supplied by the lower five paired intercostal arteries as well as the subcostal arteries.
   b. True This lies posterior to the sixth right costal cartilage.
   c. False The sympathetic trunk passes posterior to the medial arcuate ligament of each side. The crus is pierced by the greater, lesser and least splanchnic nerves.
   d. False The central tendon lies level with the lower end of the sternum, which is level with the sixth costal cartilage.
   e. True The azygos vein, the thoracic duct and the aorta all pass through the aortic opening in the diaphragm.

13. a. True This is at the thoracic inlet.
   b. False The arch of the aorta lies completely within the superior mediastinum. The plane dividing the superior and inferior mediastina lies just inferior to the level of the arch of the aorta, opposite the lower border of the fourth thoracic vertebra, and the manubriosternal junction.
   c. False It passes posterior to the right border of the sternum.
   d. False It is mainly on the right, which accords with the fact that the veins which have the potential for much expansion are on the right. The arteries are on the left, and although under greater pressure than the veins, do not expand greatly in volume. It is also the case that the spread of tumours and exudates into the superior mediastinum will be on the right for the same reasons.
   e. False It is posterior to the second right costal cartilage.

14. The trachea:
   a.   Has a length of about 15 cm.
   b.   Has a nerve supply from the vagus which is solely sensory.
   c.   Bifurcates at the level of the sternal angle.
   d.   Begins at the level of the second cervical vertebra.
   e.   Receives arterial blood from the superior thyroid artery.

15. The thymus:
   a.   Develops from the third pharyngeal pouch.
   b.   Contains Hassalblad's corpuscles.
   c.   Is the only component of the anterior mediastinum.
   d.   Derives its arterial supply from the internal thoracic artery.
   e.   Contains no nerve fibres.

14. a. True   This is about 6 in, for those who prefer imperial measures!

    b. False   Although part of the innervation provided by the vagus is sensory, vagal fibres are also secretor motor to the tracheal glands.

    c. True   This is a major landmark in the mediastinum. At this level the trachea bifurcates and the thoracic duct crosses from the right to the left. It also demarcates the lowest point of the arch of the aorta and the lowest point of the body of the fourth thoracic vertebra. Also at this level, the second costal cartilage articulates with the manubriosternal joint. A horizontal plane passing through the sternal angle separates the superior and inferior mediastina.

    d. False   It is the sixth cervical vertebra which provides this landmark.

    e. False   The superior thyroid artery mainly supplies the thyroid gland. It is the inferior thyroid artery which supplies the trachea. The venous blood drains via the brachiocephalic vein, whilst lymph follows a path back to deep cervical nodes.

15. a. True   This accounts for the epithelial component of the thymus; the lymphoid cells migrate into the structure later.

    b. False   The Hassalblad is a good – but rather expensive – photographic camera! It is Hassall's corpuscles which characterize the medulla of the thymus.

    c. False   In addition to the thymus, the anterior mediastinum also contains the sternopericardial ligaments.

    d. True   There are normally multiple branches therefrom.

    e. False   There are numerous nerve fibres present, though their function is not clear.

16. The heart:
   a. Contains musculi pectinati in the right ventricle.
   b. Has a shallow groove, the sulcus terminalis, which represents the crista terminalis on the surface of the right atrium.
   c. Receives arterial blood in its sinuatrial node by way of the left coronary artery.
   d. Drains its venous blood via the middle cardiac vein, which accompanies the posterior interventricular branch of the right coronary artery.
   e. Has surface projections of all four valves on to the sternum.

17. The posterior mediastinum contains the:
   a. Oesophagus, which in its upper part drains to the preaortic lymph nodes of the posterior mediastinum along the oesophageal arteries.
   b. Azygos vein, which passes through the caval opening of the diaphragm.
   c. Thoracic duct, which has valves at its junction with the left subclavian and left internal jugular veins.
   d. Descending thoracic aorta, which gives off four or five oesophageal arteries.
   e. Lesser and greater splanchnic nerves, which both synapse in the coeliac ganglion.

16. a. False It is trabeculae carnae in the ventricles, and musculi pectinati in the atria. Both these features are aggregations of myocardial tissue.

   b. True This demarcates the contribution of the sinus venosus in the embryonic heart and the primitive atrium.

   c. False Both right and left coronary arteries supply blood to the sinuatrial node.

   d. True The middle cardiac vein drains blood into the coronary sinus.

   e. True But note that this is not necessarily where a stethoscope would be placed to hear the sound made by the valves.

17. a. False This is the drainage for the middle part. The upper part drains via deep cervical nodes and the lower part to the coeliac nodes via lymphatics along the left gastric artery.

   b. False It makes no sense for this to be true! The azygos vein lies on the posterior thoracic wall so it would, therefore, find it difficult to access the caval opening of the diaphragm, which is further anterior. Therefore, the azygos vein passes through the aortic opening.

   c. False There are no valves in this part of the duct.

   d. True The oesophagus also receives arterial blood from the inferior thyroid and left gastric arteries.

   e. True Their targets, however, are spread throughout the abdomen. The least splanchnic nerve synapses in the renal ganglion and its fibres pass to the kidneys.

18. With regard to the lung:
  a. There are 10 bronchopulmonary segments in the right and 12 in the left lung.
  b. Its lymphatic drainage is to hilar nodes and thence directly to the thoracic duct.
  c. There is rich anastomosis between the pulmonary and bronchial arteries.
  d. The lowest level of the pleura which invests the lung is demarcated by the costal margin.
  e. The left primary bronchus is wider, more vertical and longer than its partner on the right.

19. The first rib:
  a. Is the flattest rib.
  b. Has a groove for the subclavian vein on its inferior surface.
  c. Has the subclavian vein crossing it posterior to the attachment of the scalenus anterior muscle.
  d. Is about half the length of the second rib.
  e. Is attached to the clavicle by means of the costoclavicular ligaments.

18. a. False There are 10 bronchopulmonary segments on either side. Five are above and five are below the oblique fissure. An *aide-mémoire* for these segments is APALM, APALM, APAIS, APALM – Apical, Posterior, Anterior, Lateral and Medial in the right upper and middle lobes, and the same again for the five segments of the right lower lobe. On the left side the five segments of the upper lobe are Apical, Posterior, Anterior, Inferior and Superior, whereas in the lower lobe it is APALM again.

  b. False Although drainage is to the hilar nodes, and hence to tracheobronchial nodes, these nodes drain into mediastinal lymph trunks, and then into the brachiocephalic veins directly, rather than into the thoracic duct.

  c. False There is no connection between the two supplies.

  d. False There is a small triangular portion of the pleura on each side which lies below the junction of the vertebral column and the 12th ribs.

  e. False It is the other way round – an important fact to remember when you are faced with a foreign body having disappeared down the airway! The right bronchus is usually also the one down which the anaesthetist's endotracheal tube is sometimes erroneously introduced.

19. a. True It is also the shortest and most rounded rib.

  b. False There are three structures which leave grooves on the *superior* surface of the first rib. They are the subclavian artery, vein and the lower trunk of the brachial plexus.

  c. False The subclavian vein crosses anterior to the scalenus anterior muscle, whereas the artery passes posterior to it.

  d. True See also question 10 on thorax for some more amazing facts about the ribs!

  e. True The costoclavicular ligaments are very strong. A powerful force applied to this area will break the clavicle, but the costoclavicular attachment remains intact.

Abdomen

1. **The blood supply of the stomach:**
    a. Is derived entirely from the coeliac trunk.
    b. Includes the left gastroepiploic artery, which arises from the splenic artery.
    c. Includes the right gastric artery, which arises from the gastroduodenal artery, and supplies the right side of the lesser curvature.
    d. Is very rich in numerous anastomoses.
    e. Includes a branch from the common hepatic artery which runs behind the first part of the duodenum.

2. **The external oblique muscle:**
    a. Arises by six digitations from the lower six ribs.
    b. Interdigitates with the fibres of serratus anterior and latissimus dorsi at its origin.
    c. Has a free posterior border.
    d. Has a free lower aponeurotic border.
    e. Has its fibres running downwards and forwards.

1. a. True   This is via its three branches – the left gastric, the splenic and the common hepatic artery.
   b. True   It supplies the left part of the greater curvature.
   c. False The right gastric artery usually arises directly from the common hepatic artery but it does supply the lesser curvature, anastomosing with the left gastric artery.
   d. True   A characteristic of the gastrointestinal tract.
   e. True   This is the gastroduodenal artery which, in addition to supplying the stomach, supplies the duodenum and indirectly the pancreas via the superior pancreaticoduodenal artery. The importance of the gastroduodenal artery is its anterior relationship with the first part of the duodenum. Ulcers in the latter can erode through the wall of the duodenum and involve the artery, giving rise to serious haemorrhage. Note that there is no gastroduodenal vein.

2. a. False It arises by eight digitations from the lower eight ribs.
   b. True   Its upper four slips interdigitate with the lower digitations of serratus anterior, and its four lower slips interdigitate with the fibres of latissimus dorsi.
   c. True   This is the anterior border of the lumbar triangle.
   d. False The lower aponeurotic border is the only one of the three borders of the external oblique muscle which is not free.
   e. True   An easy way to remember this is that the fibres of external oblique run in the same direction as the fingers of the hand placed in a waistcoat pocket.

3. **The rectus abdominis muscle:**
   a. Arises via two heads from the symphysis pubis and the pubic crest.
   b. Is supplied by the lower five intercostal nerves.
   c. Is attached to the fifth, sixth and seventh costal cartilages and the xiphisternum.
   d. Is a powerful flexor of the vertebral column.
   e. Plays a role in defecation and parturition.

4. **The inferior mesenteric artery:**
   a. Arises at the level of L$_4$ vertebra.
   b. Supplies the alimentary canal from the distal third of the transverse colon to the upper third of the anal canal.
   c. Is much larger than the superior mesenteric artery as it supplies a larger portion of the intestinal tract.
   d. Lies on the right psoas muscle.
   e. Crosses the pelvic brim at the level of the bifurcation of the left common iliac artery.

5. **There are a number of features which allow distinction between the large and small intestine, including:**
   a. The taenia coli of the large intestine, which are aggregates of circular smooth muscle.
   b. The appendices epiploicae of the large intestine, which have no blood supply.
   c. The haustrations of the large intestine, which are caused by the contractions of both layers of intramural smooth muscle.
   d. Peyer's patches, which occur in both small and large intestine.
   e. The enteric nervous system, which is principally present only in the large intestine.

3. a. True These are the medial and lateral heads of rectus abdominis.
   b. True It is supplied by the ventral rami of T_7–T_{12}.
   c. True It is attached in three layers from the fifth to seventh costal cartilages and the xiphisternum.
   d. True It acts on the lower thoracic and lumbar parts.
   e. True The two recti, along with the other anterolateral abdominal wall muscles and the diaphragm, compress the abdomen, increasing the intra-abdominal pressure, thereby facilitating defecation, micturition and parturition.

4. a. False It arises at the level of L_3. The aorta enters the abdomen at T_{12}, gives off the coeliac artery at L_1, the superior mesenteric artery at L_2, the inferior mesenteric artery at L_3, and divides at L_4.
   b. True These are the structures derived from the embryonic hindgut, which are supplied by the inferior mesenteric artery.
   c. False The reverse is true.
   d. False It lies on the *left* psoas muscle.
   e. True It lies in close proximity to the ureter at this site.

5. a. False Although the taenia coli are aggregations of smooth muscle in the large but not small intestine, they are of the outer, longitudinal muscle fibres. The circular layer is inside the longitudinal layer.
   b. False Appendices epiploicae are features only of the large intestine, but they do of course have a blood supply, and are not therefore to be pulled off during the course of abdominal surgery!
   c. False The presence of the haustrations in the large intestine is mainly due to the taenia coli (the longitudinal smooth muscle) as they are shorter in length than the bowel wall itself.
   d. False Peyer's patches are groups of unencapsulated lymphoid tissue found only in the ileum.
   e. False The enteric nervous system is present throughout the gastrointestinal tract and is responsible for the control of peristalsis, and of other functions. It is supplied by the autonomic nervous system, and is considered to be a separate system in its own right, with more neurons than the spinal cord!

6. **The superior mesenteric artery:**
   a. Arises at about the level of L_1.
   b. Has no branches which supply the large intestine.
   c. Does not supply the jejunum by its first branch.
   d. Emerges from the substance of the pancreas.
   e. Supplies the transverse colon by its last branch.

6. a. True   It arises about 1 cm inferior to the origin of the
coeliac artery.

b. False The superior mesenteric artery supplies the large
intestine through its right and middle colic branches.
Remember that this is via the marginal artery which
passes on the inner border of the colon, and thus
provides an anastomotic route for blood to reach all
parts of the colon, whether originally from the
superior or inferior mesenteric arteries.

c. True   The first branch of the superior mesenteric artery is
the inferior pancreaticoduodenal artery which, as its
name suggests, supplies the pancreas and duodenum.

d. True   In the embryo the pancreas develops from a dorsal
and a ventral bud. The artery passes forwards just
inferior to the larger dorsal bud. The smaller
ventral bud migrates around the foregut and comes
to lie posterior to the artery, thus it appears as
though the artery arises from within the substance
of the pancreas.

e. True   This is via the middle colic artery, which supplies
the transverse colon via the marginal artery. The
more distal parts of the colon are supplied by the
left colic branch of the inferior mesenteric artery.

7. **In the rectum:**
   a. The superior rectal artery supplies mainly the rectum and upper half of the anal canal.
   b. There are no taenia coli.
   c. The peritoneum covers its middle third.
   d. The anorectal junction is demarcated by the level of the urogenital diaphragm.
   e. Storage of faeces does not normally occur.

7. a. True The lower half of the anal canal is supplied by the
             inferior rectal artery which arises from the
             pudendal artery. There is, however, some limited
             anastomosis between the two which can be
             bolstered by the variably present middle rectal
             artery, a direct branch of the internal iliac artery.
    b. True The outer longitudinal layer of smooth-muscle
             fibres which comprise the three taenia coli of the
             sigmoid colon diverge to pass on to the anterior
             and posterior surfaces of the rectum, thus there are
             no taenia coli in the rectum.
    c. True But only on its anterior surface. There is no
             peritoneum on the lateral or posterior surfaces.
             In the upper third of the rectum, peritoneum covers
             the anterior and lateral surfaces. There is no
             peritoneum over the inferior third of the rectum,
             or anal canal.
    d. False The demarcation is the pelvic diaphragm, the
             so-called puborectalis fibres, the sling of which
             causes the perineal flexure – the demarcation of the
             anorectal junction. This sling is one of the factors
             maintaining continence.
    e. True The rectum is in reality a sense organ, which
             detects pressure from flatus, thus stimulating the
             desire to defecate. Only in the very constipated or
             at postmortem are faeces found in the rectum.

8. The liver:
   a. Is invested over its whole surface by peritoneum.
   b. Is connected to the anterior abdominal wall by the ligamentum venosum.
   c. Is supplied by the anterior gastric nerve.
   d. Is held in position by the peritoneal ligaments with which it is associated.
   e. Has physiological lobes which differ from its anatomical lobes.

8. a. False There is no peritoneal investment over the bare
area of the liver, and on the superior surface there
is no peritoneum where the latter is reflected on to
the undersurface of the diaphragm.

    b. False The ligamentum teres joins the liver to the anterior
abdominal wall. This represents the left umbilical
vein which brought oxygenated blood to the liver in
the fetus. This blood bypassed the hepatic
circulation by way of the ductus venosus, on the
visceral surface of the liver, which after birth
fibroses and becomes the ligamentum venosum.

    c. True The anterior gastric nerve also supplies the anterior
surface of the stomach, and passes up to the liver
in the free border of the lesser omentum.

    d. False The major factor which maintains the position of
the liver is the presence of the hepatic veins which
drain directly into the inferior vena cava. The
peritoneal ligaments are not strong enough to be a
major factor.

    e. True The physiological lobes make complete functional
sense, since they reflect the arterial and hepatic
portal supply to the two halves of the liver,
demarcated on the surface by a line passing
between the fundus of the gall bladder and the
inferior vena cava. The anatomical lobes, which
roughly correspond to the position of the
ligamentum teres, make no functional sense at all!

9. **The prevertebral plexus:**
   a. Contains nerve fibres from the vagus, sympathetic and pelvic splanchnic nerves.
   b. Divides at the level of the fourth sacral vertebra.
   c. Receives preganglionic sympathetic fibres via the four lumbar splanchnic nerves.
   d. Receives the thoracic splanchnic nerves and contains the ganglia in which the latter synapse.
   e. Contains mixed motor and sensory nerve fibres.

9. a. True The pelvic splanchnic nerves pass superiorly in the inferior hypogastric nerves.

 b. False Division occurs at the level of the fourth lumbar vertebra.

 c. True There are usually four lumbar splanchnic nerves, the preganglionic fibres of which have arisen in the lowest part of the thoracolumbar outflow of the sympathetic system. They pass from the upper lumbar segments of the spinal cord into the paravertebral chain of ganglia without synapsing, to enter the prevertebral plexus and synapse in one of its ganglia.

 d. True The main ganglia are the coeliac, superior mesenteric and inferior mesenteric, though there are smaller ones dispersed amongst the nerve fibres throughout the plexus.

 e. True The motor fibres supply smooth muscle and glands of the gastrointestinal tract, as well as smooth muscle in the vasculature of the abdominal viscera. Sensory nerve fibres arising from the abdominal viscera pass through the plexus to the central nervous system, having travelled with either the sympathetic or parasympathetic nerves from the viscera. Their cell bodies lie in dorsal root ganglia.

10. With regard to the pancreas:
  a. Its venous drainage is via the gastrosplenic vein.
  b. The congenital malformation known as annular pancreas arises because of malrotation of the ventral bud of the pancreas.
  c. It is supplied by arterial blood via the coeliac, superior mesenteric and splenic arteries.
  d. The tip of the tail lies in the gastrosplenic ligament.
  e. The bile duct is sometimes embedded within its substance.

10. a. False There is no such vein! Venous drainage is via the
tributaries of the hepatic portal vein, and these
veins largely follow the arterial pattern. Note,
however, that there is also no gastroduodenal vein.

   b. True Some authorities claim that the ventral bud of the
pancreas splits into two and these two portions of
pancreatic tissue migrate separately; the right
portion migrates normally, whilst the left portion
migrates in the opposite direction. This accounts
for the fact that the duodenum can become
surrounded by pancreatic tissue which could
ultimately lead to obstruction.

   c. True The superior pancreaticoduodenal artery arises
from the gastroduodenal artery (from the common
hepatic, a branch of the coeliac axis), the inferior
pancreaticoduodenal artery is the first branch of the
superior mesenteric artery, and these two vessels
principally supply the head of the pancreas. The
splenic artery supplies the body of the pancreas via
the so-called arteria pancreatica magna.

   d. False The tip of the pancreas lies in the *lienorenal
ligament*. The importance of the latter is that it
provides the route by which branches of the splenic
artery are able to supply the stomach, i.e. the short
gastric arteries and the right gastroepiploic. The
latter also supplies the greater omentum, and
anastomoses with its colleague, the left
gastroepiploic, which is a branch of the
gastroduodenal artery.

   e. True Sometimes the bile duct makes just a groove in the
posterior surface of the head of the pancreas, but
often it is embedded in its substance. A tumour of
the head of the pancreas often causes jaundice due
to biliary obstruction.

11. The spleen:
- a. Does not project any further forwards than the mid axillary line.
- b. Lies in the left hypochondrium.
- c. Is invested by the peritoneal derivatives of the dorsal mesogastrium.
- d. When enlarged, its long axis extends down and forwards along the side of the 10th rib.
- e. Forms part of the boundary of the lesser sac.

11. a. True If the spleen enlarges, it does so downwards and forwards, along the long axis of the 10th rib.

b. True This abdominal region is so named because its contents lie beneath the lower costal elements (see d).

c. True The derivatives of the dorsal mesogastrium are the greater omentum, and, in relation to the spleen, the gastrosplenic and lienorenal ligaments.

d. True Its anterior border projects out beyond the costal margin, where it may be palpable in splenomegaly. It is useful to remember certain facts about the spleen, even in these non-imperial days: it measures $1 \times 3 \times 5$ in, weighs 7 oz and lies between the ninth and 11th ribs.

e. True The left boundary of the lesser sac is made by the angle of the gastrosplenic and lienorenal ligaments.

12. The uterus:

    a.   Is covered by peritoneum only on its fundus.

    b.   Is held in place by ligaments attached to the cervix.

    c.   Normally lies in such a position that it is said to be retroverted and retroflexed.

    d.   Has the important peritoneal relation of the rectouterine pouch.

    e.   Has no nerve supply.

12. a. False The peritoneum covers the fundus and part of the body. From the urinary bladder, peritoneum ascends over the anterior surface of the bladder, making a fold, the uterovesical pouch, between the two viscera. This peritoneum also is reflected on to the posterior fornix of the vagina, from whence it is reflected superiorly on to the rectum and sacrum. Laterally, peritoneum passes to the wall of the pelvis as the broad ligament in the medial four-fifths and as the infundibulopelvic ligament in the lateral one-fifth. The ovarian arteries gain access to the ovary via the infundibulopelvic ligaments.

b. True Derived from the endopelvic fascia are the three principal ligamentous supports of the uterus: the transverse cervical, uterosacral and pubocervical ligaments. The round and broad ligaments of the uterus are not sufficiently strong to be considered supporters of the uterus.

c. False The normal uterus is anteverted and anteflexed.

d. True The rectouterine pouch, formerly known as the pouch of Douglas, is also an important posterior relation of the upper part of the vagina. Consequently, it became known as the abortionist's pouch since instruments introduced into the vagina to abort the fetus occasionally went astray and pierced the peritoneum, as they failed to enter the cervical canal. The danger of this was the possibility of causing peritonitis.

e. False The uterus is supplied by autonomic nerve fibres, though their function is unclear. Adrenergic nerves are subject to functional and structural degeneration during pregnancy, so they may be more concerned with vasculature control than reproductive function.

13. The ovary:
    a. Is covered by the germinal epithelium from which ova are derived.
    b. Is attached to the infundibulopelvic ligament.
    c. Achieves its adult position by migrating along the path of the paramesonephric duct.
    d. Is supplied only by the ovarian artery.
    e. Refers its pain along the distribution of the obturator nerve.

14. The inguinal canal:
    a. Is on average about 15 cm in length.
    b. Is formed on its anterior surface by the aponeurosis of the internal oblique muscle.
    c. Is formed posteriorly by the conjoint tendon and the fascia transversalis.
    d. Is formed inferiorly by the lateral half of the inguinal ligament.
    e. Does not contain the genitofemoral nerve in the female.

13. a. False Whilst the ovary is invested by the germinal epithelium, ova are not derived from it, as previously and erroneously thought. Primordial germ cells make their way from the yolk sac to the future ovary.

b. False The ovary is attached by means of the mesovarium to the posterior surface of the upper part of the broad ligament.

c. False The ovary migrates along the path of the gubernaculum. The remnants of the gubernaculum form the round ligaments of the ovary and uterus.

d. True This is a reflection of the high abdominal position of the ovary in its early development when it received the ovarian artery at the level of the renal arteries. The ovarian artery itself, however, also supplies part of the uterus, and anastomoses with the uterine artery.

e. True This is because the parietal peritoneum, against which the ovary lies, is supplied by the obturator nerve. The main cutaneous distribution of the obturator nerve is the medial surface of the thigh.

14. a. False The canal is about 4 cm in length.

b. False The anterior border of the canal is formed by the aponeurosis of the external oblique muscle.

c. True The conjoint tendon is formed by the fused common insertion of the internal oblique and transversus muscles on to the pubic crest.

d. False The whole of the inguinal ligament forms the floor of the canal.

e. False Although the genitofemoral nerve is not an important nerve in the female, nevertheless it traverses the canal, accompanying the round ligament, and supplying skin in the upper medial part of the thigh.

15. The spermatic cord:
   a. Has two layers of fascia.
   b. Is formed at the deep inguinal ring.
   c. Contains three arteries and two nerves.
   d. Contains a branch of the pudendal nerve.
   e. Does not contain the lymphatics of the scrotum.

16. Of the surface markings of the abdomen:
   a. The transpyloric plane lies at the same level as the subcostal plane.
   b. The umbilicus lies at the level of the junction of the third and fourth lumbar vertebrae.
   c. The fundus of the gall bladder is approximately at the same level as the hila of the kidneys.
   d. The neck of the pancreas is at the same level as the fundus of the gall bladder.
   e. The duodenojejunal flexure lies at the level of the subcostal plane.

15. a. False The spermatic cord has *three* layers of fascia – the external spermatic fascia, derived from the external oblique muscle; the cremasteric fascia derived from the internal oblique muscle and which contains the muscle fibres of the cremaster muscle; and the internal spermatic fascia, derived from the transversalis fascia.

  b. False It is formed at the superficial inguinal ring; proximal to this ring insufficient layers will have been acquired to form the cord fully.

  c. True The three arteries are the testicular, cremasteric (from the inferior epigastric artery) and the artery of the ductus deferens (from the inferior vesical artery). The two nerves are the genital branch of the genitofemoral nerve and autonomic nerves.

  d. False The pudendal nerve supplies the perineum and has no branches within the spermatic cord. It is the *genitofemoral* nerve which lies within the spermatic cord.

  e. True The lymphatics from the scrotum do not ascend in the spermatic cord, but in the superficial fascia to the superficial inguinal lymph nodes.

16. a. False These two planes are not the same. The transpyloric plane is defined as the imaginary horizontal line which passes through the pylorus of the stomach, lying midway between the pubic symphysis and the xiphisternum. The subcostal plane lies at the lowest point of the costal margin, opposite the upper part of the third lumbar vertebra. The transpyloric plane lies opposite the first lumbar vertebra.

  b. True Whilst this is the case in the normal, slim, adult, in infants and in those individuals with protruding, pendulous abdomens, the umbilicus may be somewhat lower.

  c. False Whilst the fundus of the gall bladder is on the transpyloric plane, the right hilum of the kidney is just below, and the left hilum of the kidney is just above the transpyloric plane.

  d. True Of course the body and tail of the pancreas lie successively higher, as they pass laterally across the abdominal wall.

  e. False The duodenojejunal flexure lies on the transpyloric plane.

17. The anterolateral abdominal wall muscles:
   a.   Above the costal margin, form the anterior rectus sheath, which comprises the external and internal oblique aponeuroses.
   b.   And the anterior rectus sheath consist of only the transversalis fascia below the arcuate line.
   c.   Contain the superior and inferior epigastric arteries.
   d.   Have their nerve supply from the seventh to 11th intercostal nerves only.
   e.   Are separated by the linea alba in the midline, which is not bloodless.

18. Regarding the lymphatic drainage of the abdomen:
   a.   The lesser curvature of the stomach drains to the suprapancreatic nodes.
   b.   The kidneys drain directly into para-aortic nodes.
   c.   Lymphatics draining the intestine tend to follow the pattern of the venous drainage.
   d.   The spleen has no lymph drainage.
   e.   Lymph from the small intestine passes directly into the intestinal trunk.

17. a. False Above the costal margin the anterior layer of the rectus sheath consists only of the external oblique aponeurosis.

b. False The anterior rectus sheath, below the arcuate line, is formed by the aponeuroses of the external and internal oblique, and transversus muscles. The transversalis fascia forms the only posterior boundary to the rectus muscles.

c. True There is an anastomosis between the superior epigastric artery (from the internal thoracic artery) and the inferior epigastric (from the external iliac artery).

d. False The nerve supply of the anterolateral abdominal wall muscles is from the seventh to 11th intercostal, subcostal (12th thoracic spinal nerve) and the iliohypogastric and ilioinguinal nerves.

e. True The linea alba is almost all fibrous tissue, but nevertheless, it does have some blood vessels in it. Notwithstanding the presence of these vessels, the linea alba is a useful structure in which to make a midline abdominal incision. Apart from the little bleeding that will occur, it does not damage the rectus sheath, particularly above the umbilicus.

18. a. False The lesser curvature partly drains to lymphatics along the left gastric artery to reach the coeliac nodes, and partly to nodes along the course of the right gastric artery.

b. True These nodes are situated at about the level of the second lumbar vertebra, the level at which the renal arteries arise.

c. False The lymph pattern is arranged in three orders: first, in nodes near the intestine; second, in nodes in the mesentery; and third, in nodes which are arranged around the origins of the superior or inferior mesenteric arteries. The course taken by the lymph vessels is along the supplying *arteries*.

d. False The spleen drains via nodes at the hilum to retropancreatic nodes, and thence to the coeliac group around the origin of the same-named artery.

e. False Lymph in lacteals passes through the three orders of lymph nodes which drain the intestine.

19. The autonomic nerve supply to the gastrointestinal tract:
    a. Is derived solely from the vagus and sympathetics.
    b. Does not supply the visceral peritoneum.
    c. Does not arise from the inferior hypogastric plexus.
    d. Does not supply gut epithelia.
    e. Includes sympathetics from usually four lumbar splanchnic nerves.

20. With regard to the superficial fascia of the abdomen:
    a. The membranous layer of the fascia of the abdominal wall is part of the hypodermis.
    b. The lumbar fascia has three layers.
    c. The fascia transversalis is adherent to parietal peritoneum.
    d. Fascia lata and the membranous fascia of the abdominal wall are in the same tissue plane.
    e. The posterior layer of the rectus sheath is an example of the membranous layer of fascia.

19. a. False Parasympathetic supply is also derived from the pelvic splanchnic nerves (root value S_{2-4}).

   b. False Visceral peritoneum receives an autonomic nerve supply, in common with the rest of the viscus it invests.

   c. False Parasympathetic nerve fibres from the pelvic splanchnic nerves pass through the inferior hypogastric plexus *en route* to the prevertebral plexus for distribution to the distal colon. Sympathetic nerve fibres from the lower lumbar splanchnic nerves may gain access to the colon via this route.

   d. False Afferent autonomics have been demonstrated in close proximity to the gut epithelium, normally subjacent to the basement membrane.

   e. True The lumbar splanchnic nerves are an oft-forgotten category of preganglionic sympathetic nerve fibres.

20. a. False The hypodermis is the layer deep to the dermis of the skin. This is synonymous with the superficial fascia, the fat layer around our well-fed bodies! The deep fascia is the membranous layer.

   b. True The anterior layer of the lumbar fascia lies anterior to psoas major, the middle layer separates the latter from the quadratus lumborum muscle, and the posterior layer covers the erector spinae muscle layer.

   c. True In general, there are areas where the parietal peritoneum is very firmly adherent to the fascia of the abdominal wall, e.g. posterior to the linea alba. In some areas there is a much looser arrangement, i.e. where peritoneum is reflected over the surface of the urinary bladder on to the inner surface of the anterior abdominal wall.

   d. True Both these are examples of deep fasciae.

   e. False The rectus sheath is aponeurotic tissue, i.e. a muscle insertion.

21. With regard to the peritoneum:
   a. The posterior boundary of the aditus to the lesser sac is the caudate lobe of the liver.
   b. The serosa passing from the lesser curvature of the stomach to the visceral surface of the liver is derived from the septum transversum.
   c. The serosa on the undersurface of the diaphragm is more absorptive than elsewhere.
   d. The paraduodenal fossae are extraperitoneal.
   e. The hepatorenal pouch is the right posterior subphrenic space.

22. The duodenum:
   a. Has a first part which passes superiorly to the left and posteriorly, making contact with the liver.
   b. Has the common bile duct passing posterior to its first part.
   c. Has posterior relationships in its third part with the inferior vena cava, abdominal aorta and the common bile duct.
   d. Receives arterial blood from the superior pancreaticoduodenal, inferior pancreaticoduodenal and retroduodenal arteries, the latter arising from the superior mesenteric artery.
   e. Has an interior which is thrown into folds throughout the length of the duodenum.

21. a. False The posterior boundary of the aditus is the posterior abdominal wall. The caudate lobe of the liver is the superior boundary.

b. True This is the derivative of the ventral mesogastrium. The peritoneum passing from the liver to the stomach, the peritoneal investments of the liver, the connective tissue of the liver, and the central tendon of the diaphragm also arise from the septum transversum.

c. False All areas of the peritoneum are equally absorptive.

d. False These fossae are lined by peritoneum.

e. True In the recumbent position this is the lowest point of the peritoneal cavity, and effusions may accumulate in this area, with the possibility of abscess formation.

22. a. True This relationship may result in duodenal ulcers eroding the liver.

b. True It passes at a point 2.5 cm from the pyloroduodenal junction.

c. False This is illogical, since the bile duct enters the second part of the duodenum, and therefore cannot be related to the third part, though it is related to the inferior vena cava and the abdominal aorta.

d. False Although all these vessels supply the duodenum with arterial blood, the retroduodenal artery arises from the *gastroduodenal artery*. This is a branch of the common hepatic artery, which arises from the coeliac trunk, not the superior mesenteric artery. The splenic artery also supplies the duodenum.

e. False Most of the interior of the duodenum is thrown into folds known as plicae circulares, but the first part is smooth.

23. The kidney:
   a. Is fixed in its position on the posterior abdominal wall.
   b. Has as its anterior relation on the right the third part of the duodenum.
   c. Has arteries which supply its five segments and in which there are frequent anastomoses.
   d. Receives an afferent nerve supply by way of the sympathetic nerves that arise from the 12th thoracic to second lumbar spinal cord segments.
   e. Hilum is about 5 cm from the abdominal aorta.

24. In the abdominal wall:
   a. The iliohypogastric nerve pierces the external oblique aponeurosis just below the superficial inguinal ring.
   b. The subcostal nerve is only cutaneous.
   c. The lumbar veins communicate with the azygous system.
   d. The thoracolumbar fascia is attached to the transverse processes of the lumbar vertebrae.
   e. The ligamentum flavum lies on the anterior surface of the bodies of the lumbar vertebrae.

23. a. False The kidney moves with respiration.
    b. False It is the second part of the duodenum which has this relationship. The third part lying across the midline could not be related to either kidney!
    c. False There are normally five segmental vessels supplying the kidney, but these are virtually end-arteries.
    d. True These fibres carry pain impulses.
    e. True In relation to the inferior vena cava, though, the right kidney is much closer than the left.

24. a. False The iliohypogastric nerve pierces the aponeurosis just *above* the superficial inguinal ring.
    b. False The subcostal nerve supplies the muscles of the anterolateral abdominal wall as well as skin. It is not, however, part of the lumbar plexus, being the ventral ramus of the 12th thoracic spinal nerve.
    c. True This communication can open up sufficiently to allow blood to return to the heart in cases of caval or portal obstruction. There are communications with the veins draining the lower limbs too.
    d. True This particular part of the fascia is the middle lamella.
    e. False The ligamentum flavum connects adjacent laminae and lies *posterior* to the bodies of the lumbar vertebrae. In general, all the ligaments of the lumbar spine are thicker and stronger than elsewhere, consistent with the increased load-bearing of the lumbar spine.

25. The surface markings of the abdomen include:
a. The highest point of the iliac crest, which lies at the level of the intervertebral disc, between the fourth and fifth lumbar vertebrae.
b. The lowest level of the costal margin, which lies at the level of the third lumbar vertebra.
c. The fundus of the gall bladder, which lies at the lateral border of the right rectus abdominis muscle just below the tip of the ninth costal cartilage.
d. The pancreatic neck, which lies at the level of the first lumbar vertebra.
e. The pylorus of the stomach, which lies on a level about two lumbar vertebrae lower in the erect position.

26. With respect to the biliary apparatus:
a. The arterial supply most commonly arises from the right hepatic artery.
b. The parasympathetic nerve supply is from the posterior vagal trunk.
c. The gall bladder normally holds a volume of 10 ml.
d. The average length of the common bile duct is 10 cm.
e. The bile duct lies anterior and to the left of the other structures in the free border of the lesser omentum.

27. The suprarenal gland:
a. Is tetrahedral in shape.
b. On the right lies between the inferior vena cava and the median arcuate ligament.
c. Receives arterial blood from its own named vessel, and from the inferior phrenic and lumbar arteries.
d. Has a cortex which is derived from the neural crest.
e. On the left is a direct relation of the pancreas.

25. a. True This is a point of great clinical significance as this is considered a safe level to perform a lumbar puncture, the spinal cord ending level with the second lumbar vertebra.

    b. True This is at the 10th costal cartilage.

    c. True This is on the transpyloric plane.

    d. True This is the level of the transpyloric plane.

    e. True The pylorus also lies at a lower level in females compared to males.

26. a. True This is, however, the site of considerable variation, a point of surgical relevance.

    b. False It is from the anterior vagal trunk, which is logical since it is the anterior trunk which passes via the free border of the lesser omentum to supply the liver. The posterior trunk passes posteriorly to enter the prevertebral plexus.

    c. True It will also hold a normal maximum of 50 ml!

    d. True The cystic and hepatic ducts are normally about 4 cm in length.

    e. False It lies anterior and to the right. The hepatic artery lies anterior and to the left, whilst the portal vein is posterior.

27. a. False The right gland is pyramidal and the left is crescentic in shape.

    b. False It lies between the inferior vena cava and the right crus of the diaphragm.

    c. False The lumbar arteries do not supply the suprarenal gland. It is supplied by the suprarenal, renal and inferior phrenic arteries.

    d. False It is the medulla which is derived from the neural crest. The phaeochromocytes are the chromaffin cells, identified by histologists of old by the ability of these cells to take up chromium salts. The cortex is derived from mesoderm.

    e. True The left gland is crossed by the pancreas which is passing up to the hilum of the spleen.

28. **The transverse colon:**
    a. Is in direct contact with the anterior abdominal wall.
    b. Has the convexity of the greater curvature of the stomach lying within its concavity.
    c. Has less numerous and smaller appendices epiploicae than elsewhere in the colon.
    d. May reach down as far as the pelvic brim.
    e. Terminates at the left colic flexure at the level of the 10th costal cartilage.

29. **The ureter:**
    a. Is narrowest at the pelvi–ureteric junction, at the point where it crosses the common iliac vessels, and where it enters the urinary bladder.
    b. Has two layers of smooth muscle.
    c. Begins at a point opposite the *ninth* costal cartilage.
    d. Derives its blood supply from the renal artery, vesical arteries, gonadal artery and the lumbar arteries.
    e. Undergoes peristalsis.

28. a. True   Note that the transverse mesocolon is adherent to the greater omentum which, of course, is reflected on to the posterior abdominal wall.

    b. True   This is also because of its relationship with the greater omentum.

    c. False They are larger and more numerous than elsewhere.

    d. True   A point to be appreciated in interpretation of barium enemas.

    e. False It is at the level of the *eighth* costal cartilage.

29. a. True   It is at these points that a ureteric calculus may become arrested.

    b. False It has *three* layers of smooth muscle: an inner circular, middle longitudinal and outer circular layer. These layers are really spirals of muscle fibres, and the layers tend to intermingle somewhat. In the lower part of the ureter the outer circular layer may be absent.

    c. True   It passes down to the level of the bifurcation of the common iliac artery. This point is easy to find since it lies halfway on a line between the pubic symphysis and the anterior superior iliac spine.

    d. False The lumbar arteries do not supply the ureter. All the other three do, and there is sometimes supply from the common iliac artery.

    e. True   This wave is thought to originate from pacemakers in the renal minor calyces. It is a useful means of identifying the ureter at surgery as peristalsis can be induced by light mechanical stimulation.

30. The appendix:
  a. In the majority of cases hangs down below the caecum.
  b. Receives arterial blood from the anterior caecal artery.
  c. May be over 20 cm long.
  d. Has a wider lumen in infants.
  e. Has a base which is said to lie at the point where the three taenia coli meet.

31. With regard to the abdominal aorta:
  a. On the right, in its upper part, it is related above to the cisterna chyli, thoracic duct, azygos vein and right crus of the diaphragm.
  b. On the left, it is related above to the median arcuate ligament, and left coeliac ganglion.
  c. Posteriorly, it is related to the upper four lumbar vertebrae, and all the lumbar arteries and veins.
  d. It is crossed by the neck of the pancreas.
  e. When the abdominal wall is relaxed the pulsations of the aorta may be visible just above its bifurcation.

30. a. True The position is quite variable. In the majority of cases it lies behind the caecum. However, various surveys present conflicting data.

b. False It receives arterial blood by way of the appendicular artery which is a branch of the posterior caecal, which arises from the ileocolic branch of the superior mesenteric artery.

c. True It is longer in children, and shorter in adults. A particularly long appendix can contact a variety of other abdominal organs and thus there is potential for spread of inflammation.

d. True In the elderly the lumen is often obliterated. Even though it is wider in infants, it is still narrow and therefore subject to faecal impactions and resulting infection.

e. True The actual surface marking for the base of the appendix is at a point just inferior and medial to the intersection of the transtubercular and the right lateral vertical plane.

31. a. True The right crus of the diaphragm separates the aorta from the inferior vena cava (and right coeliac ganglion).

b. False These relations cannot lie to the left of the aorta because the median arcuate ligament lies in the midline.

c. False It is related only to the third and fourth (sometimes the second) lumbar veins.

d. False It is crossed by the body of the pancreas.

e. True This will be easier to spot in a thin individual, and lies at the level of the fourth lumbar vertebra. These pulsations may also be visible in the epigastric region.

32. The common iliac artery:
  a. Is about 8 cm long.
  b. Passes obliquely across the fourth and fifth lumbar vertebrae.
  c. Has the sympathetic trunk lying posterior to it and anterior to the vertebrae.
  d. Lies midway on a line between the anterior superior iliac spine and the pubic symphysis.
  e. Has no other branches aside from its termination in the external and internal iliac arteries.

33. With regard to the branches of the coeliac trunk:
  a. The right gastric artery is the smallest branch.
  b. In later fetal life the common hepatic artery is the largest branch of the coeliac trunk.
  c. The short gastric arteries arise from the splenic artery and are two or three in number.
  d. A common variation of the origin of the hepatic artery includes an origin from the superior mesenteric artery.
  e. May have more than three branches.

34. The small intestine:
  a. Has a mesentery whose root is about 15 cm long and is attached from the left side of the first lumbar vertebra to the right sacroiliac joint.
  b. Has a mesentery whose root crosses successively the horizontal part of the duodenum, abdominal aorta, inferior vena cava and right psoas major muscle.
  c. Is thicker-walled in the jejunum.
  d. Has an average distance from the root of the mesentery to the intestinal border of about 20 cm.
  e. Distal to the duodenojejunal flexure is jejunum in its proximal two-thirds.

32. a. False On the right it is about 5 cm long, but on the left it is about 4 cm long.
  b. True The fourth and fifth lumbar vertebrae are the posterior relations of both common iliac arteries.
  c. True The sympathetic trunk lies between the lumbar vertebrae and the common iliac arteries.
  d. True Though note that it arises one-third of the way along this line.
  e. False The common iliac artery gives off small branches to the peritoneum, ureter and psoas major muscle. Occasionally, the iliolumbar and accessory renal arteries arise from the common iliac artery.

33. a. False The left gastric artery is the smallest coeliac branch.
  b. True This size difference continues into postnatal life.
  c. False There are usually five to seven branches.
  d. True Amongst other variations in the arrangement of the hepatic artery are accessory right and left hepatic arteries. The former most frequently arises from the left gastric and the latter from the superior mesenteric artery.
  e. True Whilst it is true that there are only three main branches, it may also give rise to one or both inferior phrenic arteries.

34. a. False The mesentery starts at the level of the *second* lumbar vertebra.
  b. False The mesentery also crosses the right ureter, after it passes the inferior vena cava.
  c. True It is also more vascular, and is therefore redder in appearance. Its villi are also larger, it has more plicae circulares but it has fewer unencapsulated lymphoid follicles than the ileum.
  d. True On average the distance from root to intestinal border is said to be 20 cm, though this can be greater, particularly at intermediate positions along the length of the small intestine.
  e. False It is jejunum in its proximal two-fifths. The junction between the jejunum and the ileum, however, is not distinct. There is a gradual histological transition from one to the other. The most characteristic parts of the jejunum and ileum are at their beginning and end respectively.

35. The stomach:
 a. Has a cardiac orifice which opens at a point just posterior to the right ninth costal cartilage.
 b. Has a pylorus with a sphincter which is thickened longitudinal smooth muscle.
 c. Has a mean capacity which may be as much as 1500 ml.
 d. Has its fundus level with the left fourth intercostal space.
 e. Is completely invested by peritoneum.

36. The liver:
 a. Has a right lobe which contributes to all surfaces.
 b. Has caudate and quadrate lobes which occupy the entire liver substance from anterior to posterior surfaces.
 c. Can extend into the left hypochondrium as far as the left lateral line.
 d. Has no impression on it for the oesophagus.
 e. Has no fibrous capsule intervening between the liver itself and the visceral peritoneum covering it.

37. With regard to the kidneys:
 a. The anterior surface of the right kidney includes a colic area.
 b. The anterior surface of the left kidney does not include a colic area.
 c. The suprarenal, pancreatic and colic areas of the left kidney are devoid of peritoneum.
 d. The perirenal fascia is a synonym for renal fascia.
 e. The inferior poles may extend to the level of the first sacral vertebra.

35. a. False The cardiac orifice lies just behind the right *seventh* costal cartilage.
    b. False It is circular smooth muscle.
    c. True In infants, however, it has a volume of only 30 ml.
    d. False It lies level with the left fifth intercostal space. In males this is just below the nipple, though varying with respiration. It is possible, therefore, in a stab wound to this area to involve the fundus of the stomach.
    e. True The peritoneum is derived from the ventral and dorsal mesogastria.

36. a. True The right lobe is much larger than the left.
    b. False These two smaller lobes are demarcated by shallow grooves and thus they are only present on the posterior and inferior surfaces and therefore do not occupy the entire liver substance from anterior to posterior.
    c. True The left lateral line is the vertical plane which is also known as the mid clavicular line. It passes through the mid inguinal point.
    d. False There is a groove on the left lobe made by the oesophagus as the oesophagus passes towards the stomach, which produces the gastric impression on the visceral surface of the liver.
    e. False There is such a capsule, formerly known as Glisson's capsule.

37. a. True This area is located in the lower half of the right kidney, from its lateral border to a more medial strip related to the duodenum.
    b. False The colic area overlies the lower lateral half of the left kidney.
    c. True Note that these areas are adjacent to each other.
    d. False The two are different. The perirenal fascia is fat which surrounds the kidney; the renal fascia is fibrous connective tissue which surrounds the fat.
    e. False The inferior poles descend to a point no more than 2.5 cm above the iliac crests, which are at the level of the fourth lumbar vertebra. Of course, the right kidney is always lower than the left because of the liver.

38. **Of the anterolateral muscles of the abdominal walls:**
    a. The external oblique muscle attaches to the lower eight ribs only.
    b. The internal oblique muscle attaches to the lower three ribs.
    c. The transversus abdominis muscle arises from the lower six ribs.
    d. The rectus abdominis muscle is inserted into the fifth to seventh ribs.
    e. The pyramidalis muscle lies anterior to the lower part of the internal oblique muscle.

39. **The somatic nerves of the lumbar plexus include:**
    a. The iliohypogastric, which pierces the external oblique aponeurosis just below the superficial inguinal ring.
    b. The ilioinguinal, which supplies the skin of the labium majus.
    c. The genital branch of the genitofemoral nerve, which also supplies skin in the labium majus.
    d. The femoral branch of the genitofemoral, which passes posterior to the inguinal ligament.
    e. The lateral femoral cutaneous nerve, which does not supply skin other than that of the thigh.

38. a. True It arises from the outer surfaces of these ribs.
   b. True The lower borders of the lower three ribs (and their costal cartilages) are attachments for the internal oblique muscle, though other attachments include the lumbar fascia, anterior two-thirds of the iliac crest and the lateral two-thirds of the inguinal ligament.
   c. True The transversus muscle also has attachments to the costal cartilages of those ribs.
   d. False It is to the costal cartilages of those ribs that the rectus abdominis muscle is attached.
   e. False When present, this small muscle lies anterior to the lower part of rectus abdominis.

39. a. False The iliohypogastric nerve normally pierces the aponeurosis about 3 cm *above* the superficial inguinal ring.
   b. True The ilioinguinal nerve also supplies the skin of the proximomedial part of the thigh, and that of the root of the penis or the mons pubis.
   c. True In males it ends by supplying the skin of the scrotum and the cremaster muscle.
   d. True It then continues to supply skin on the anterior to the upper part of the femoral triangle. In so doing, with its genital partner, it facilitates the cremasteric reflex.
   e. False This nerve may supply the gluteal region, in addition to its distribution over the lateral part of the thigh.

40. As regards the veins in the vertebral column:
    a.   The external vertebral venous plexus is most well developed in the lumbar region.
    b.   The basivertebral veins enter the bone of the vertebral column.
    c.   They contain non-return valves.
    d.   There are extensive interconnections between the external and internal vertebral venous plexa.
    e.   They communicate with segmental venous drainage.

41. With regard to the lymphatic drainage of the abdomen:
    a.   There are no lymphatics in the pancreatic islets.
    b.   The thoracic duct does not lie in the abdomen.
    c.   The intestinal trunks receive lymph from the preaortic nodes.
    d.   The pararectal nodes drain the rectum and upper half of the anal canal.
    e.   Drainage from the kidney is in three parts.

40. a. False It is most developed in the cervical region.
   b. True This is partly why bone metastases may be found in cancers of the pelvic viscera.
   c. True This is another factor explaining the frequency of metastases from tumours in the pelvic region.
   d. True This interconnecting network of veins also has communications with the azygous system and may permit blood to return to the heart if there is an obstruction in the inferior vena cava, or the hepatic portal vein. In any event, any increase in intra-abdominal pressure can reverse the direction of the blood within these vessels.
   e. True Thus lumbar and posterior intercostal veins communicate with the plexa.

41. a. True The drainage from the exocrine portion passes to pancreaticoduodenal nodes, from whence it passes to preaortic nodes. There is no lymphatic drainage from the endocrine portion.
   b. False The duct extends from the level of the second lumbar vertebra before passing into the thorax via the aortic opening of the diaphragm.
   c. False It is the other way round! The preaortic nodes receive lymph from the intestinal trunks.
   d. True From the pararectal nodes lymph passes on to the group of nodes around the origin of the superior rectal artery, and thereafter to nodes around the origin of the inferior mesenteric artery.
   e. True One around the renal tubules, one under the capsule of the kidney and a third in the perirenal fat. From these plexa lymph drains to lateral aortic nodes.

42. With regard to the nerve supply of peritoneum:
   a. That from the central tendon region of the diaphragm passes via the phrenic nerve.
   b. That from the peripheral parts of the diaphragm passes via the fifth and sixth intercostal nerves.
   c. There is no afferent supply from visceral peritoneum.
   d. Parietal and visceral layers both respond to the same stimuli.
   e. There is no motor supply to peritoneum.

43. The ascending colon:
   a. Extends superiorly into the right (splenic) flexure.
   b. Lies on the iliac fascia.
   c. Is supplied by the ileocolic and right colic arteries.
   d. Gives rise to the vermiform appendix which occupies the left iliac fossa.
   e. May be relatively short.

42. a. True   Direct mechanical stimulation of this point causes pain to be referred to the tip of the shoulder, because the root value of the phrenic nerve is shared by the supraclavicular nerves which supply skin over this region.

  b. False   It is via the seventh to 12th intercostal nerves and the first lumbar nerves.

  c. False   There *is* an afferent nerve supply from the visceral peritoneum. It responds to pressure stimuli.

  d. False   Parietal peritoneum responds to painful stimuli such as trauma, whereas visceral peritoneum responds to increases in intraluminal pressure.

  e. False   Though not extensive, the blood vessels within the visceral peritoneum require vasomotor fibres.

43. a. False   The ascending colon extends superiorly into the right colic (*hepatic*) flexure.

  b. True   The ascending colon does indeed lie on the iliac fascia, as well as partly on the lumbar fascia. The parietal peritoneum, which covers the side and front of the colon at these points, is thus reflected from the abdominal wall on medial and lateral sides, thus forming the medial and lateral paracolic gutters.

  c. True   It is supplied by the ileocolic and right colic arteries, though these two vessels feed into the so-called marginal artery which is an anastomotic artery from which blood passes to the colon itself. Note that the ileocolic artery also supplies the terminal ileum, but that both arteries arise from the superior mesenteric artery, the artery of the embryonic midgut.

  d. False   It is the *caecum* which gives rise to the vermiform appendix, though the latter does occupy the left iliac fossa.

  e. True   In these circumstances the ascending colon may hardly exist, and a subhepatic caecum brings the caecum near to the liver. This is accounted for on embryological grounds by the failure of the ascending colon to lengthen during development.

44. The sigmoid colon:
a. Lies anterior to the third lumbar vertebral segment.
b. Is incompletely invested by peritoneum.
c. Is constant in length.
d. Has a mesocolon whose apex of attachment is related to the ureter, whose lumen is widest at this point.
e. Is supplied by sigmoidal branches of the descending left colic artery.

45. The caecum:
a. Contains the ileocolic valve.
b. Is supplied by anterior and posterior caecal arteries.
c. Lies on the posterior abdominal wall overlying the obturator nerve.
d. Has three taenia coli which converge at the ileocaecal junction.
e. Gives rise to the vermiform appendix which may receive its blood supply (the anterior caecal artery) at the base of the appendix.

44. a. False The sigmoid colon commences at a point which lies opposite the third sacral vertebral segment.

   b. True It is incompletely invested by the peritoneum of the sigmoid mesocolon, whose root on the abdominal wall occupies an inverted V shape.

   c. False It is quite variable in length and may sometimes rise quite some distance out of the pelvis. It is a store for faeces, which is the main reason why it needs length, and hence requires to be slung from a mesentery.

   d. False The apex of the mesocolon is related to the ureter, but it is the lumen of the latter which is *reduced* at that point.

   e. False The sigmoidal arteries arise as direct branches from the inferior mesenteric artery, the artery of the embryonic hindgut.

45. a. False It contains the *ileocaecal valve*. This structure guards the orifice of the caecum, preventing reflux of colonic contents into the caecum. The term valve, however, is a misnomer since no valvular structure exists, but simply a thickening of the circular smooth-muscle fibres which encircle the terminal ileum.

   b. True It is supplied by anterior and posterior caecal arteries which themselves arise from the ileocolic artery.

   c. False It does lie on the posterior abdominal wall but overlying the *femoral* nerve.

   d. False The converging taenia coli demarcate the base of the *vermiform appendix*.

   e. False There are two untruths in this question. First, it is the posterior caecal artery which supplies the appendix, and second, the appendicular artery (often reputed to be the most commonly ligated artery in surgery) enters the appendix some short distance from its tip, often via the variably present mesoappendix.

46. Meckel's diverticulum:
    a.   Is present in about 15% of the population.
    b.   May be up to 60 cm in length.
    c.   May contain gastric mucosa.
    d.   Lies at the point of attachment of the vitellointestinal duct.
    e.   Lies at the point of attachment of the vitelline duct.

46. a. False It is present in about 2% of the population.
    b. False It may be up to 5 cm in length; however, it usually lies about 60 cm from the ileocaecal junction.
    c. True For this reason it may become ulcerated, and mimic the pain induced in the early stages of appendicitis – pain in the umbilical region.
    d. True The duct lies at the point in the embryo where there was continuation of the midgut and the yolk sac. In the adult this connection becomes fibrous and usually disappears. It can, however, persist, and a number of difficulties can arise. These include the duct remaining patent, cyst formation and intestinal obstruction caused by intestine becoming caught by it.
    e. True The vitelline duct is synonymous with the vitellointestinal duct!

47. The lesser sac:
  a. Lies posterior to the stomach.
  b. Has an aditus which has free communication with the hepatorenal pouch.
  c. Is relatively much smaller in the fetus.
  d. Is functionless.
  e. Can only be entered by making a slit in the greater omentum, just inferior to the greater curvature of the stomach.

47. a. True It lies posterior to the stomach, as well as part of the caudate lobe of the liver. In this location it is the upper extension of the lesser sac, the left posterior subphrenic space. The lesser sac may also be found in between the diverging layers of the greater omentum, but only for 2 cm or so below the greater curvature of the stomach.

    b. False This is rubbish! The aditus is in free communication with the greater sac, a small part of which is the hepatorenal pouch, though this latter structure is some distance from the lesser sac, being the right posterior subphrenic space.

    c. False It is relatively much *larger* in the fetus because it passes inferiorly between the diverging layers of the greater omentum, to the free inferior border of the latter.

    d. False Some might say that it is functionless, though those kinds of arguments are always fatuous. Most likely it is an expansion space for a full stomach. The more phlegmatic might say that it simply results from the rotation of the stomach and duodenum.

    e. False Again, this is rubbish! The aditus is the only entry point, and this is located behind the free border of the lesser omentum, above the roof of the first part of the duodenum, under the caudate lobe of the liver, and in contact with the posterior abdominal wall at the point where it is traversed by the inferior vena cava.

Pelvis and perineum

1. **In the pelvic floor the musculature:**
   a. Consists of levator ani and piriformis.
   b. Includes the puborectalis which forms a sling around the anorectal junction and merges with the superficial part of the external anal sphincter.
   c. Has the perineal branch of the fourth sacral nerve passing to the perineum between piriformis and iliococcygeus.
   d. Has the inferior rectal nerve supplying the major part of levator ani from its superior surface.
   e. Has the nerves of the sacral plexus lying posterior to the pelvic fascia.

2. **With regard to the rectum:**
   a. The superior rectal artery supplies only the rectum.
   b. The superior rectal artery has three branches which pass into the wall of the anal columns. It is the left branch of the artery which divides again into anterior and posterior branches to give a total of three branches.
   c. There is rich anastomosis between the branches of the middle rectal and inferior rectal arteries.
   d. The lymph drainage of the rectum includes lymphatics which travel with the median sacral artery.
   e. There are no non-return valves in the veins draining the rectum.

1. a. False The musculature of the pelvic floor consists of levator ani and coccygeus.
   b. False The puborectalis merges with the *deep* part of the external anal sphincter.
   c. False This nerve passes between coccygeus and iliococcygeus supplying both muscles on their superior surface.
   d. False This nerve supplies the muscles of the pelvic floor from their inferior surface.
   e. True In the pelvis the nerves lie posterior and the blood vessels lie anterior to the fascia.

2. a. False It supplies the rectum and the anal canal as far distally as the point where the mucous membrane changes its character from columnar to keratinized stratified squamous epithelium.
   b. False It is the right branch of the superior rectal artery which divides into two further branches.
   c. False No significant anastomoses occur between all three rectal arteries – superior, middle and inferior – which supply the rectum and anal canal.
   d. False The principal drainage is via lymphatics which lie along the superior and middle rectal arteries and thence to the preaortic nodes.
   e. True This is the principal reason why blood can pass either via the vertebral venous plexus to the inferior vena cava or hepatic portal vein tributaries. This constitutes a potential route for spread of infective emboli or metastatic cells.

3. The urinary bladder:
   a. Is lined by stratified squamous epithelium.
   b. Has lymphatics which drain to nodes alongside the internal iliac artery.
   c. Has a trigone whose epithelium is endoderm-derived.
   d. Has a medial umbilical ligament arising from its apex.
   e. Lies anterior to the anal canal in the male.

4. The prostate:
   a. Is roughly the size and shape of a tangerine.
   b. Has an anteriorly placed longitudinal ridge called the urethral ridge.
   c. Has an opening at the apex of the urethral crest, the prostatic utricle, which is a derivative of the urogenital sinus.
   d. Has a fascia which is continuous with its capsule.
   e. Is supplied by blood from the inferior vesical and middle rectal arteries, which enter the prostate medially at its junction with the urinary bladder.

3. a. False It is lined by transitional epithelium.
    b. True The main lymph drainage is via lymphatics along
             the superior and inferior vesical arteries, and thence
             to nodes lying on the lateral wall of the pelvis
             alongside the internal iliac artery.
    c. False It is derived from the mesoderm, whereas the rest
             of the epithelium is derived from endoderm.
             Consequently, it is of different nerve sensitivities.
    d. False It is the *median* umbilical ligament which arises
             from the apex of the urinary bladder. It is the
             allantois in the embryo which is an unimportant
             structure in humans, though in some animals it is
             involved in the formation of the placenta. It is,
             nevertheless, of clinical significance in relation to its
             patency leading to sinus or cyst formation.
    e. False It is the rectum which is a posterior relation of the
             urinary bladder in the male. In females, the uterus
             and upper part of the vagina are related to the
             urinary bladder.

4. a. False It is normally the size and shape of a chestnut.
             Of course, particularly in middle-aged and elderly
             men, it can enlarge significantly.
    b. False The urethral crest is posteriorly placed.
    c. False The prostatic utricle is derived from the
             paramesonephric ducts, which in females give rise
             to the uterus, and uterine tubes. It is of no
             significance.
    d. False The fascia and capsule are separate from each
             other, in a space occupied by the prostatic venous
             plexus. The latter communicates with the vertebral
             venous plexus, which explains the observation that
             prostatic cancers can metastasize to bone of the
             vertebral column.
    e. False The arteries enter the prostate laterally.

5. **The uterus:**
   a. Has lymphatics which pass with the uterine artery to the internal iliac nodes.
   b. Has a round ligament, which is the major factor which stabilizes the position of the organ.
   c. Has a cervical canal, which is characterized by interdigitations called arbor vitae.
   d. Is covered by the peritoneum of the round ligament, which constitutes the route by which nerves and blood vessels from the pelvic wall gain direct access to the organ.
   e. Has the uterine tubes entering its fundus.

6. **The pelvic vessels include:**
   a. The iliolumbar artery which passes superiorly as it leaves the pelvis, posterior to the lumbosacral trunk.
   b. The superior gluteal artery which leaves the pelvis via the lesser sciatic foramen.
   c. The obturator artery which emerges from the pelvis through the greater sciatic notch and re-enters it through the lesser.
   d. The internal pudendal artery which leaves the pelvis via the greater sciatic foramen to lie inferior to the piriformis muscle.
   e. The lateral sacral artery which lies posterior to the roots of the sacral plexus.

5. a. True However, some lymph can pass along the round ligament to superficial inguinal nodes. Cancer of the body of the uterus must be excluded when finding a lump in the area of these nodes.

    b. False The major stabilizing factor is the ligaments attaching the uterine cervix to the pelvic walls, i.e. the transverse cervical, the uterosacral and the pubocervical.

    c. True Not to be confused with the arbor vitae of the cerebellum! In the uterus they are said to reduce the chance of infection spreading into the peritoneal cavity.

    d. False The route by which nerves and blood vessels gain access from the lateral pelvic wall is first by the lateral one-fifth of peritoneum, known as the infundibulopelvic ligament; they then cross into the *broad* ligament, which is the medial four-fifths of this same peritoneal covering.

    e. False The uterine tube enters the uterus at the junction of the body and fundus, at the so-called cornua.

6. a. False The iliolumbar artery is a branch of the posterior division of the internal iliac artery and passes *anterior* to the lumbosacral trunk. It supplies musculature of the pelvic walls, including the iliopsoas and erector spinae muscles.

    b. False The superior gluteal artery passes out of the pelvis through the greater sciatic foramen before it supplies the gluteus medius and minimus, as well as cutaneous branches overlying the buttock and taking part in the trochanteric anastomosis.

    c. False This is rubbish! The obturator artery leaves the pelvis by passing through the obturator foramen. The pudendal artery leaves via the greater and enters via the lesser sciatic foramina.

    d. True The internal pudendal artery does indeed pass out of the greater sciatic foramen and lies inferior to piriformis before it supplies structures within the perineum.

    e. False The lateral sacral artery lies *anterior* to the roots of the sacral plexus, and obeys the rule that nerves lie posterior to the pelvic fascia and vessels lie anterior to it.

7. **The sacral plexus:**
   a. Gives rise to a posterior cutaneous nerve of the thigh, which is formed from the roots of the first to fourth sacral spinal nerves.
   b. Has pelvic splanchnic nerves which pass towards the inferior hypogastric nerves via the ventral rami of the second to fourth sacral spinal nerves.
   c. Has the nerve to obturator internus which also supplies the inferior gemellus muscle.
   d. Has the nerve to quadratus femoris which passes out of the pelvis posterior to the sciatic nerve.
   e. Gives rise to the lumbosacral trunk which lies superior to the ala of the sacrum as it passes on to join the plexus.

8. **In the anal triangle of the perineum:**
   a. Is contained the anal canal whose sphincter is composed solely of voluntary muscle.
   b. The sides of the anal canal are formed by the sacrospinous ligaments.
   c. There are different contents in the two sexes.
   d. Lies the ischioanal fossa which contains only fat.
   e. The sensory nerve supply to the skin is derived from the fourth and fifth lumbar spinal nerves.

7.   a. False It is formed by the roots of the second and third sacral spinal nerves.
    b. True These are the parasympathetic nerves of the pelvis.
    c. False The nerve to obturator internus supplies the superior gemellus. The inferior gemellus muscle is supplied by the nerve to quadratus femoris.
    d. False The nerve passes out of the pelvis anterior to the sciatic nerve.
    e. False The fourth and fifth lumbar spinal nerves emerge from the lumbar plexus and are considered to be the lumbar root of the lumbosacral trunk.

8.   a. False Whilst the external anal sphincter is of voluntary striated muscle, the internal sphincter is derived from longitudinal smooth muscle.
    b. False It is the sacrotuberous ligaments which form the sides of the triangle.
    c. False This is an occasion when one can truly say that there is no difference between the sexes (though one might argue that the pudendal nerve is different)!
    d. False The inferior rectal nerve and vessels pass across the fossa (previously, and illogically, called the ischiorectal fossa). These structures may potentially be damaged during drainage of an ischioanal fossa abscess.
    e. False It is the fourth *sacral* spinal nerve which supplies this area. The fourth and fifth lumbar spinal nerves supply skin in the leg.

9. In the urogenital triangle of the perineum:
   a. The superficial perineal space has the perineal membrane as its superior border.
   b. The superficial perineal space contains only fat and vessels.
   c. The deep perineal space contains the deep transverse perineal muscle.
   d. The deep perineal space is also known as the urogenital diaphragm.
   e. The sphincter urethrae muscle is innervated by the perineal branch of the pudendal nerve, and has a root value of S_4.

10. Regarding the penis:
   a. The artery of its bulb is a branch of the perineal artery.
   b. The deep artery of the penis gives rise to the helicine arteries.
   c. The dorsal arteries of the penis pass to the glans, where they anastomose with branches of the artery of the bulb.
   d. The urethra is contained within the corpus cavernosus.
   e. The superficial dorsal vein of the penis lies outside the fascia penis.

9. a. False The perineal membrane is the inferior border of the space.
  b. False Whilst it contains fat and vessels, it also contains the ischiocavernosus and bulbospongiosus muscles and their nerves. It is traversed by the urethra in both sexes and by the vagina in the female.
  c. True The fibres of this muscle are interwoven with those of the sphincter urethrae muscle around the urethra.
  d. False The urogenital diaphragm consists of the deep perineal space plus the perineal membrane and the superior layer of fascia of the urogenital diaphragm (which overlies the deep transverse perineal muscle of the deep space).
  e. False It is innervated by the perineal branch of the pudendal nerve, which has a root value of $S_{2,3}$. The perineal branch of S_4 supplies the external anal sphincter (along with the inferior rectal nerve, which has a root value of $S_{3,4}$).

10. a. False It is a branch of the internal pudendal artery.
  b. True It is these vessels which supply the cavernous tissue of the penis, which is involved in the mechanism of erection.
  c. True There are two dorsal arteries and they are enclosed by the fascia penis.
  d. False The penile portion of the urethra is contained within the corpus spongiosum; the membranous part lies within the urogenital diaphragm, and the prostatic part within the prostate.
  e. True It drains into the superficial external pudendal veins, which drain into the femoral vein at the saphenous opening.

11. The joints of the pelvis include:

a. The iliolumbar ligaments, which are attached to the ala of the sacrum and pass to the iliac crest.

b. The pubic symphysis, which can sometimes develop a synovial cavity.

c. The posterior sacroiliac ligaments, which join the sacrum and the ilium, but are rather weak.

d. The sacrococcygeal joint, which permits flexion and extension and lateral flexion.

e. The coccyx, whose triangular form arises from the two bones which fuse to make up this final bone of the vertebral column.

12. With regard to nerve supply:

a. The mucous membrane of the penile urethra is supplied by the deep dorsal penile nerve.

b. The skin of the clitoris is supplied by the dorsal nerve which arises from the pudendal nerve.

c. The ilioinguinal nerve supplies the anterior two-thirds of the scrotum.

d. The posterior one-third of the scrotum is supplied by the dorsal rami of the 5th sacral spinal nerve.

e. The sacrospinalis muscle is a member of the deep layer of the erector spinae group and is supplied by the dorsal rami of the sacral spinal nerves.

11. a. False They are attached to the fifth lumbar vertebra.
 b. False It can sometimes develop a fluid-filled cavity,
  arising from tissue fluid, but it is not lined by
  synovium.
 c. False It is the anterior sacroiliac ligaments which are
  weak, not the posterior sacroiliac ligaments, which
  are very strong. Their strength holds together the
  pelvic ring, which would otherwise be disrupted by
  the weight of the upper part of the body.
 d. False No side-to-side movement is permitted. Strictly
  speaking, humans cannot wag their tails!
 e. False Phylogenetically the coccyx is related to the tail of
  other animals; it forms as four pieces which fuse
  together. It is not, itself, however, a joint of the
  pelvis, though it does articulate with the sacrum at
  the sacrococcygeal joint.

12. a. False It is supplied by the perineal branch of the
  pudendal nerve. There is no deep dorsal nerve.
  The dorsal nerve supplies the skin of the penis.
 b. True This is the equivalent of the dorsal nerve of the
  penis.
 c. False It supplies the anterior one-third.
 d. False The posterolateral two-thirds of the scrotal skin are
  supplied by scrotal branches of the perineal nerve
  (S_3), and the perineal branch of the posterior
  cutaneous nerve of the thigh (S_2). The anterior
  one-third of the scrotal skin is supplied by the
  ilioinguinal nerve (L_1). The former is derived from
  the sacral plexus and the latter from the lumbar
  plexus. This demarcation is due to the axial line
  which separates the posterolateral two-thirds of the
  scrotal skin from the anteromedial one-third.
 e. False Sacrospinalis is supplied by sacral spinal nerve
  dorsal rami; however, it lies in the *superficial* layer
  of the erector spinae.

13. With regard to the vestibule of the vagina:
a. The bulb contains erectile tissue which passes into the clitoris.
b. The prepuce of the clitoris is derived from the labia minora.
c. The vestibular glands moisten the labia majora.
d. The vagina has a sphincter formed by the bulbospongiosus muscle, as well as the pubovaginalis (sphincter vaginalis) muscle.
e. The vestibular glands lie superficial to the bulbospongiosus muscle.

14. With regard to the ischioanal fossa:
a. The anococcygeal body receives fibres from the sacrotuberous ligament.
b. The perineal body lies deep to the puborectalis muscle.
c. The pudendal canal lies between the lesser sciatic foramen and the posterior boundary of the perineal membrane.
d. It can extend as far as the back of the pubis, deep to the urogenital diaphragm.
e. The inferior rectal nerve supplies no part of the rectum.

15. Regarding the external anal sphincter:
a. The subcutaneous part is not attached to bone.
b. The superficial part is supplied by the perineal branch of the fourth sacral spinal nerve.
c. The deep part is attached to bone.
d. It has the superficial part as its middle layer lying between the subcutaneous and deep parts.
e. It is paralysed following injury to the pudendal nerve.

13. a. True In particular it passes into the glans of the clitoris.
     b. True The labia minora also form a ventral frenulum for the glans.
     c. False They moisten the vaginal orifice.
     d. True The two are not continuous however.
     e. False They lie deep to the bulbospongiosus muscle.

14. a. False It receives interdigitating fibres from the iliococcygeus and pubococcygeus muscles.
     b. True This body, together with the anococcygeal body, strengthens the midline of the floor of the perineum, the latter being potentially weakened by the passage of the urethra and anorectal junction in both sexes, and the vagina in the female.
     c. True By this means the perineum is supplied by the pudendal nerve, and its branch, the perineal nerve. The canal itself consists of thickened fascia of the obturator internus muscle, which forms the lateral wall of the ischioanal fossa.
     d. True There is, however, but little communication between the two sides.
     e. True It supplies structures associated with the anal canal only.

15. a. True It is attached to surrounding fascia, and itself is a ring-like structure.
     b. True This is a branch of the pudendal nerve.
     c. False It is not attached to bone, and is a ring-like muscle though its posterior fibres blend with those of puborectalis.
     d. True This is the correct disposition. Do not be confused by the misleading names of the three layers.
     e. True This can occur during overzealous evacuation of an ischioanal fossa abscess.

16. With regard to the penis:
   a. It contains the urethra which is lined throughout by transitional epithelium.
   b. The urethra is vertical in cross-section, in line with the external meatus.
   c. It is supplied throughout its length by the perineal nerve.
   d. Lymph drains to the superficial inguinal lymph nodes only.
   e. The three corpora of the penis are invested by the tunica vaginalis.

17. The scrotum:
   a. Contains the dartos muscle, which is supplied by the perineal branch of the fourth sacral spinal nerve.
   b. Contains the testes and spermatic cords.
   c. Is supplied by the superficial and deep external pudendal arteries which are branches of the external iliac arteries.
   d. Is drained by the superficial and deep external pudendal veins which drain into the obturator vein.
   e. Contains no fat.

16. a. False The epithelium lining the portion of the urethra
before the prostatic urethra is transitional.
Thereafter, it becomes pseudostratified or stratified
columnar. At the tip of the external meatus it
becomes keratinized.
   b. False It is horizontal in cross-section, whereas the meatus
is vertical, hence the spiral stream that doth flow!
   c. True The nerve enters by piercing the corpus spongiosum
of the bulb of the penis.
   d. False It drains to both superficial and deep inguinal
lymph nodes.
   e. False They are invested by the tunica albuginea. The
tunica vaginalis invests the testis.

17. a. True These are sympathetic fibres which supply this
smooth muscle. This musculature is said to be part
of the panniculus carnosus which enables the skin
of horses and cattle to shudder.
   b. True The coverings of the testes are continuous with the
spermatic cord fascial coverings.
   c. False The superficial and deep external pudendal arteries
are branches of the internal iliac arteries. The
scrotum is also supplied by the internal pudendal
artery posteriorly.
   d. False They drain into the great saphenous vein and
thence to the femoral vein, via the saphenous
opening.
   e. True The subcutaneous layer of the scrotum contains no
fat; instead it contains the dartos muscle.

18. **In the testis:**
    a. The ductuli afferentes lead from the rete testis to the head of the epididymis.
    b. The ductus deferens lies medial to the epididymis.
    c. Each seminiferous tubule is about 60 cm in length.
    d. There are sympathetic nerves arising from the first and second lumbar spinal cord segments.
    e. There is no parasympathetic nerve supply.

19. **The internal iliac artery:**
    a. Supplies the rectum and anal canal via its superior and middle rectal branches.
    b. Gives rise to branches to the gluteal region which pass above and below piriformis.
    c. Gives rise to the inferior epigastric artery which sometimes has an aberrant obturator artery as one of its branches.
    d. Supplies the lower part of the ureter via its branches.
    e. Arises from the bifurcation of the common iliac artery at the level of L_4.

18. a. False It is the ductuli *efferentes* which number about
12–15, and pass superiorly to the head of the
epididymis. There are no *afferent* ductules in the
testis.

b. True The narrow space lying between the two is the
sinus of the epididymis.

c. True These tubules are highly convoluted.

d. False They arise from the 10th thoracic spinal cord
segments, in accord with the embryological origin
of the testis.

e. True This is logical since there is no thoracic or lumbar
parasympathetic outflow. The vagus nerve does not
pass sufficiently inferior to reach the testis, and the
pelvic splanchnic nerves do not leave the pelvis.

19. a. False The superior rectal artery is the terminal branch of
the inferior mesenteric artery. The internal iliac
supplies the rectum and anal canal via the middle
rectal artery and the inferior rectal artery, which is
a branch of the internal pudendal artery.

b. True These are the superior and inferior gluteal arteries,
thus named according to their relationship to the
piriformis muscle.

c. False The inferior epigastric artery arises from the
external iliac artery, though it can give rise to an
aberrant obturator artery.

d. True This is via its superior and inferior vesical
branches. The branches of the internal iliac artery
in the male can be remembered by means of the
mnemonic: Such Is Life, Some Inherit Money,
Others Inherit Insanity. (From the posterior
division – Superior gluteal, Iliolumbar and Lateral
sacral; from the anterior division – Superior vesical,
Inferior vesical, Middle rectal, Obturator, Internal
pudendal, Inferior gluteal.)

e. False The common iliac artery bifurcates at a lower level,
anterior to the sacroiliac joint, level with the
lumbosacral intervertebral disc. The abdominal
aorta bifurcates at the level of L_4.

20. The lumbar plexus:
    a. Provides the nerve supply of the entire lower limb.
    b. Gives rise to the femoral nerve which is derived from the anterior divisions of L_{2-4}.
    c. Gives rise to the obturator nerve which emerges from the medial aspect of psoas major muscle.
    d. Gives rise to the iliohypogastric and the ilioinguinal nerves, both of which share a root value of L_1.
    e. Gives rise to the lateral femoral cutaneous nerve (lateral cutaneous nerve of the thigh) which usually passes below or pierces the inguinal ligament.

21. The pudendal nerve:
    a. Is the main motor and sensory supply of the pelvic floor and perineum.
    b. Has a root value of S_{1-3}.
    c. Arises from three twigs which unite to form the nerve which passes between piriformis and coccygeus to reach the ischioanal fossa.
    d. Has the inferior rectal nerve as one of its branches which supplies the levator ani.
    e. Has the perineal nerve as one of its terminal branches.

20. a. False The sacral plexus is also a major contributor to the nerve supply of the lower limb. Its largest branch, the sciatic nerve, is one of the main nerves supplying the lower limb and has a root value of $L_{4,5}S_{1-3}$.

   b. False It is the obturator nerve which arises from the anterior divisions of L_{2-4}. The femoral nerve arises from the posterior divisions of L_{2-4}.

   c. True It then passes through the obturator foramen to supply the muscles of the adductor compartment.

   d. True The ilioinguinal nerve is said to be the collateral branch of the iliohypogastric nerve.

   e. True Its root value is $L_{2,3}$.

21. a. True Injury to the pudendal nerve will cause laxity in the muscles of the pelvic floor with associated incontinence.

   b. False To complete the mnemonic mentioned in Thorax question 9, $C_{3,4 \text{ and } 5}$ keeps my diaphragm alive, $S_{2,3 \text{ and } 4}$ keeps my bits off the floor.

   c. True Once it reaches the ischioanal fossa it enters the pudendal canal.

   d. True The inferior rectal nerve is also motor to the external anal sphincter. Levator ani is also supplied by the perineal branch of S_4.

   e. True The other is the dorsal nerve of the penis (clitoris).

22. The rectum:
    a. Receives its blood supply from the superior, middle and inferior rectal arteries, the superior being the main artery supplying the mucous membrane.
    b. Receives some of its blood supply from the middle rectal artery – a branch of the external iliac artery which may sometimes be absent.
    c. Receives some of its blood supply from the internal pudendal artery via the inferior rectal artery.
    d. Has a venous drainage which includes the middle rectal vein, which ultimately drains to the portal circulation.
    e. Has a lymph drainage which ultimately reaches both the inferior mesenteric and internal iliac lymph nodes.

22. a. True The superior rectal artery is the continuation of the inferior mesenteric artery and the largest of the three vessels supplying the rectum.

   b. False The middle rectal artery may sometimes be absent. However, when present, it arises from the *internal* iliac artery.

   c. True The inferior rectal also supplies the anal canal.

   d. False The middle rectal vein drains into the internal iliac vein, which is part of the systemic circulation. It is the superior rectal vein which drains into the portal circulation, and this constitutes one of the sites of portosystemic anastomosis.

   e. True The upper part of the rectum drains along the course of the superior rectal artery to the inferior mesenteric lymph nodes, whereas the lower part of the rectum drains along the course of the middle rectal artery to the internal iliac lymph nodes.

Head and neck

1. **Regarding the autonomic ganglia in the head and neck:**
   a. The sympathetic fibres to the dilator pupillae muscle arise from the Edinger–Westphal nucleus.
   b. All the four parasympathetic ganglia receive a sensory root from one of the branches of the trigeminal nerve.
   c. The lacrimal gland receives its parasympathetic fibres via the pterygopalatine ganglion.
   d. The submandibular ganglion receives its sympathetic fibres directly from the stellate ganglion.
   e. The nervus intermedius provides the parasympathetic component for both the pterygopalatine and submandibular ganglia.

2. **The facial nerve:**
   a. Exits from the skull via the jugular foramen, passes through the petrous temporal bone, and emerges from the skull through the stylomastoid foramen.
   b. Emerges from the parotid gland giving off temporal, zygomatic, buccal, mandibular and cervical branches.
   c. Is the nerve of the fourth branchial arch.
   d. Supplies the stapedius muscle.

1. a. False It is the parasympathetic fibres to the sphincter
pupillae muscle which arise from the Edinger–
Westphal nucleus. The sympathetic fibres arise from
the upper thoracic segments of the spinal cord.
 b. True The four parasympathetic ganglia are the ciliary,
pterygopalatine, submandibular and otic. They can
be remembered by the mnemonic: cats prefer sexy
owners. The ciliary receives its sensory root from
the ophthalmic branch of the trigeminal nerve, the
pterygopalatine via the maxillary branch and the
submandibular and otic ganglia receive their
sensory supply via the mandibular branch of the
trigeminal nerve.
 c. True The pterygopalatine ganglion supplies the palate,
nose and nasopharynx, paranasal sinuses, the
lacrimal gland and the labial glands in the upper lip.
 d. False The stellate ganglion is another name for the
cervicothoracic ganglion which usually results from
the fusion of the inferior cervical and the first
thoracic sympathetic ganglia. All the cranial
parasympathetic ganglia receive their sympathetic
input via the superior cervical ganglion.
 e. True The fibres are carried to the pterygopalatine
ganglion via the greater petrosal nerve and to the
submandibular ganglion via the chorda tympani.

2. a. False It passes into the internal acoustic foramen,
through the petrous temporal bone, and eventually
emerges from the stylomastoid foramen.
 b. True The branches of the facial nerve after it emerges
from the parotid gland can be remembered by
means of the mnemonic: **T**en **Z**ulus **B**ought **M**y **C**at
(**T**emporal, **Z**ygomatic, **B**uccal, **M**andibular and
Cervical). The original mnemonic has been amended
to avoid offending Zulus and animal lovers.
 c. False The facial is the nerve of the second branchial arch.
It is the superior laryngeal branch of the vagus
which is the nerve of the fourth branchial arch.
 d. True The stapedius muscle arises from the mesoderm of
the second branchial arch, and is therefore supplied
by the facial nerve, the nerve of the second
branchial arch.

3. **The paranasal air sinuses include:**
   a. The maxillary sinus, which opens into the middle meatus.
   b. The sphenoid air sinus, which lies just beneath the pineal gland.
   c. The ethmoidal air sinuses, which all open into the middle meatus.
   d. The frontal sinus, which is the only one which has developed at birth.

4. **Regarding the foramina in the base of the skull:**
   a. The middle meningeal artery passes through the foramen spinosum which lies in the sphenoid bone.
   b. The glossopharyngeal nerve passes through a foramen in the occipital bone.
   c. The spinal component of the accessory nerve passes out of the skull with the hypoglossal nerve.
   d. The foramen rotundum transmits the greater petrosal nerve.

3. a. True   All the paranasal sinuses open into the middle
               meatus except the posterior ethmoidal sinus which
               opens into the superior meatus and the sphenoidal
               air sinus which opens into the sphenoethmoidal
               recess. Note that the opening of the maxillary sinus
               lies above its lowest point. This accounts for the
               fact that paranasal sinus infection occurs most
               commonly in the maxillary sinus.
    b. False The sphenoidal air sinus lies just beneath the pituitary
               gland. This is the route for trans-sphenoidal
               hypophysectomy.
    c. False The anterior and middle ethmoidal air cells do open
               into the middle meatus; however, the posterior
               ethmoidal air cells open into the *superior* meatus.
    d. False The frontal air sinus is absent at birth. All the
               others are rudimentary except the maxillary sinus,
               which may be identifiable.

4. a. True   When this artery is damaged, it is often the source
               of bleeding in extradural haematomas.
    b. True   It passes through the jugular foramen which lies
               between the occipital and petrous temporal bones.
    c. False It passes out through the jugular foramen with the
               glossopharyngeal (IX), vagus (X) and cranial
               accessory (XI) nerves.
    d. False This is rubbish. The greater petrosal nerve passes to
               the foramen lacerum where it is joined by the deep
               petrosal nerve. They unite to form the nerve of the
               pterygoid canal and pass through it to the
               pterygopalatine ganglion. The foramen rotundum
               transmits the maxillary branch of the trigeminal
               nerve.

5. Regarding the blood supply of the brain:
    a. It is derived entirely from the internal carotid and vertebral arteries.
    b. Multiple pontine branches arise directly from the basilar artery.
    c. The anterior inferior and the superior cerebellar arteries arise from the basilar artery.
    d. The posterior communicating artery joins the middle cerebral and posterior cerebral arteries, and lies in close proximity to the oculomotor nerve.
    e. The two vertebral arteries come together to form the basilar artery on the ventral surface of the midbrain.

6. The venous drainage of the brain:
    a. Is via venous sinuses which lie between the dura and the arachnoid mater.
    b. Includes the great cerebral vein (of Galen) which drains into the cavernous sinus.
    c. Mainly leaves the skull via the sigmoid sinus, which indents the inner surface of the occipital bone.
    d. Includes the superior and inferior petrosal sinuses which drain into the superior and inferior sagittal sinuses respectively.
    e. Includes the straight sinus which drains into the transverse sinus.

7. The CSF:
    a. Is formed only by the choroid plexus of the lateral and third ventricles.
    b. Can be collected for laboratory analysis from the right lateral ventricle by means of a burr hole in the right posterior parietal or right frontal region.
    c. Passes from the third ventricle to the subarachnoid space via the foramina of Magendie and Luschka – the median and two lateral apertures.
    d. Is present in the vertebral canal down to the mid lumbar level.
    e. Is present in larger amounts in elderly patients.

5. a. True The external carotid supplies the dura, but not the brain, via the middle meningeal artery which arises from its maxillary branch.
   b. True It also has cerebellar and labyrinthine branches.
   c. True The posterior inferior cerebellar artery arises from the vertebral artery.
   d. True Aneurysms of the posterior communicating artery can compress the oculomotor nerve, causing an ipsilateral dilated pupil.
   e. False They come together on the ventral surface of the medulla.

6. a. False They are intradural venous sinuses, lying between the meningeal and endosteal layers of the dura.
   b. False The great cerebral vein (of Galen) drains into the straight sinus.
   c. True And most of it usually leaves through the right sigmoid sinus which passes through the jugular foramen, becoming the internal jugular vein.
   d. False The superior petrosal sinus drains into the sigmoid sinus, and the inferior petrosal opens into the jugular bulb.
   e. True This occurs at the confluence of sinuses.

7. a. False It is also secreted, though to a lesser extent, by the choroid plexus of the fourth ventricle, and possibly by the ependymal lining of the ventricular walls.
   b. True It can also be obtained by lumbar puncture or cisternal puncture.
   c. False It is from the fourth ventricle that it passes to the subarachnoid space.
   d. False The dural sac, which contains CSF, extends down to the midsacral level. CSF can easily be obtained by lumbar puncture at L_{4-5} level.
   e. True Cerebral atrophy inevitably occurs in older individuals, and the ventricles and subarachnoid spaces which are filled by CSF become larger.

8. The posterior triangle of the neck:
   a. Lies between sternocleidomastoid and trapezius.
   b. Contains the three cords of the brachial plexus.
   c. Contains the accessory nerve.
   d. Contains the occipital lymph nodes.
   e. Contains all three scalene muscles.

9. The strap muscles of the neck:
   a. Include sternohyoid and omohyoid which lie superficial to sternothyroid and thyrohyoid.
   b. Include the two sternohyoid muscles which diverge to allow the thyroid cartilage to protrude between them.
   c. Include the omohyoid muscle, which usually attaches to the middle third of the clavicle.
   d. Includes the omohyoid muscle, which has two bellies, both of which are innervated by branches of the ansa cervicalis.
   e. Include geniohyoid and thyrohyoid, which are innervated via the hypoglossal nerve.

8. a. True It extends from the level of the superior nuchal line down to the level of the clavicle.

b. False It is the three *trunks* of the brachial plexus which lie in the posterior triangle of the neck. The cords are in the axilla.

c. True It emerges beneath the posterior border of sternocleidomastoid, supplies it, and then passes downwards to supply the trapezius.

d. True The occipital lymph nodes lie in the apex of the posterior triangle.

e. True Splenius capitis, levator scapulae and the first digitation of serratus anterior also usually lie within the posterior triangle of the neck.

9. a. True The muscles which attach to the thyroid cartilage lie in a deeper plane to the other two infrahyoid muscles.

b. True The prominence thus produced is the Adam's apple or laryngeal prominence.

c. False It usually attaches inferiorly to the upper border of the scapula and the transverse scapular ligament.

d. True All the strap muscles of the neck are supplied segmentally from the ansa cervicalis. Do not confuse the omohyoid with the digastric muscle, which also has two bellies, each of which has a different nerve supply.

e. True The fibres however are from C_1. They have merely travelled with the hypoglossal nerve. It is therefore correct to state that all the strap muscles of the neck are innervated by the ansa cervicalis. The mylohyoid, which has a separate innervation from the mandibular nerve, is not considered to be one of the strap muscles.

10. The facial muscles:
a. Include orbicularis oculi, which is made up of a palpebral and an orbital part.
b. Have the basic function of opening and closing the facial orifices.
c. Include buccinator, which is considered to be an accessory muscle of mastication.
d. Include the orbicularis oris muscle, which is the sphincter of the lips, and the dilator muscles which insert into it in a radial manner.
e. Are all innervated by the mandibular branch of the trigeminal nerve, which is the only one of the three branches of the trigeminal nerve which carries motor fibres.

11. Sternocleidomastoid:
a. Arises via two heads.
b. Turns the head in the direction of the contracting muscle.
c. Receives its blood supply segmentally from the external carotid artery.
d. Moves the face forward when both muscles contract together.
e. Is innervated via the cranial nerve XI.

10. a. True The palpebral fibres arise from the medial palpebral ligament and insert into the lateral palpebral raphe, whereas the orbital fibres take origin from the bony orbit and circumscribe the eye. Together they close the eyelids.

    b. True This is their basic function. Facial expression is a byproduct which has evolved in the human species.

    c. True Buccinator is a muscle of facial expression, but since it returns the bolus from the cheek pouch for further mastication by the molars, it is also considered to be an accessory muscle of mastication.

    d. True It is obvious that contraction of muscles which insert radially into the sphincter will dilate it.

    e. False The mandibular branch of the trigeminal nerve is the only one of the three branches of the trigeminal nerve which carries motor fibres. However, it is motor to the muscles of mastication and not to the facial muscles. The facial muscles are innervated by the facial nerve.

11. a. True It has a manubrial head and a clavicular head.

    b. False It turns the head in the opposite direction from the contracting muscle. Feel your own!

    c. False There are no direct muscular branches from the external carotid (see Head and neck question 12). Sternocleidomastoid receives its blood supply from branches of the occipital and superior thyroid arteries – both of which arise from the external carotid.

    d. True Both muscles can be felt contracting when the head is protracted.

    e. True The fibres which innervate sternocleidomastoid arise from the upper cervical segments. They pass intracranially through the foramen magnum and exit through the jugular foramen with IX, X and XI cranial nerves. They join the accessory (XI) nerve and ultimately supply sternomastoid and trapezius.

12. The external carotid artery:
    a. Does not contribute to the blood supply of any intracranial structures.
    b. Supplies the thyroid gland via the inferior thyroid artery.
    c. Contains the carotid body within its wall.
    d. Arises at the level of the lower border of the thyroid cartilage.
    e. Crosses over the parotid gland.

13. The olfactory nerves:
    a. Are not 'true' cranial nerves.
    b. Arise from the neuroepithelium in the roof of the nose.
    c. Pass through the cribriform plate of the ethmoid bone in the form of about 20 olfactory nerve filaments.
    d. Synapse in the olfactory bulb.
    e. Converge on the thalamus before reaching the cortex.

12. a. False The middle meningeal artery arises from the maxillary artery, which is a branch of the external carotid. It is for this reason that the external carotid artery is sometimes ligated preoperatively in patients with large vascular meningiomas.

b. False It supplies the thyroid gland via the *superior* thyroid artery. The branches of the external carotid artery can be remembered by means of the mnemonic: **As She Lay Flat, Oscar's Passion Slowly Mounted** – **A**scending pharyngeal, **S**uperior thyroid, **L**ingual, **F**acial, **O**ccipital, **P**osterior auricular, **S**uperficial temporal and **M**axillary. The original mnemonic had to be altered as it would have been unlikely that we would have been able to publish this book using the traditional mnemonic! The inferior thyroid artery arises from the thyrocervical trunk, which is a branch of the first part of the subclavian artery.

c. False The carotid body lies behind the bifurcation of the common carotid artery. It functions as a chemoreceptor.

d. False It arises at the bifurcation of the common carotid artery, which is at the level of the greater horn of the hyoid bone.

e. False It lies within the substance of the parotid gland.

13. a. True This applies to both the olfactory and the optic nerves. They are both considered to be outgrowths from the central nervous system rather than true cranial nerves.

b. True This is the site of the first sensory neurons.

c. True They pierce the dura and arachnoid and relay in the olfactory bulb. In basal skull fractures involving the cribriform plate of the ethmoid bone, these filaments may be amputated, leading to anosmia.

d. True The second-order neurons are in the olfactory bulb. Their processes extend to the anterior perforated substance and the uncus.

e. False The sense of smell is a primitive function which has retained its unique arrangement, even in the more complex human central nervous system. The second-order neuron connects directly with the cortex without passing through the thalamus.

14. The optic nerve:
   a.   Is covered in pia, arachnoid and dura.
   b.   Has its nasal fibres carrying images from the temporal field of vision.
   c.   Passes through the superior orbital fissure.
   d.   Is supplied by the ophthalmic artery.

15. The oculomotor nerve:
   a.   Carries parasympathetic nerve fibres.
   b.   Passes through the superior orbital fissure.
   c.   Is responsible for the dilated pupil associated with an extradural haematoma.
   d.   Is responsible for the dilated pupil associated with aneurysms of the posterior communicating artery.

14. a. True   This is why papilloedema is seen in the optic disc in increased intracranial pressure.

b. True   It is these fibres which decussate in the optic chiasma.

c. False   It passes through the optic foramen.

d. True   This is the first branch of the internal carotid artery.

15. a. True   The parasympathetic nerve fibres carried by the oculomotor nerve arise from the accessory oculomotor nucleus (Edinger–Westphal nucleus) and are destined for the sphincter pupillae and ciliary muscles, which they reach via the ciliary ganglion (see Head and neck question 1).

b. True   The nerves which pass through the superior orbital fissure are III, IV, V_1 and VI. The oculomotor nerve (III) divides into a superior and inferior branch, and the ophthalmic nerve (V_1) divides into the lacrimal, frontal and nasociliary nerves. A useful mnemonic for the nerves which pass through the superior orbital fissure is: **Lazy French Tarts Sat Naked In Anticipation** – **L**acrimal, **F**rontal, **T**rochlear, **S**uperior oculomotor, **N**asociliary, **I**nferior oculomotor and **A**bducent.

c. True   An extradural haematoma will lead to an increase in intracranial pressure, and eventually to herniation of the supratentorial contents through the tentorial opening. This will lead to trapping of the oculomotor nerve (usually on the same side as the extradural haematoma) between the herniating uncus of the temporal lobe and the unyielding tentorium. This pressure on the oculomotor nerve will paralyse the sphincter pupillae. The pupil will therefore dilate and the light reflex will be abolished.

d. True   The oculomotor nerve lies in very close proximity to the posterior communicating artery. An aneurysm arising from the posterior communicating artery can compress the oculomotor nerve, leading to dilatation of the pupil, complete ophthalmoplegia and ptosis.

16. The inferior orbital fissure:
  a. Connects the orbit to the anterior cranial fossa.
  b. Transmits the maxillary branch of the trigeminal nerve.
  c. Lies between the greater and lesser wings of the sphenoid bone.
  d. Transmits the zygomatic nerve, which is a branch of the facial nerve.
  e. Transmits the infraorbital artery, which is a branch of the facial artery.

16. a. False The inferior orbital fissure connects the orbit to the infratemporal and pterygopalatine fossae. The *superior* orbital fissure connects the orbit and the *middle* cranial fossa.

b. True The maxillary branch of the trigeminal nerve leaves the middle cranial fossa via the foramen rotundum and enters the pterygopalatine fossa. It then enters the orbit via the inferior orbital fissure. It eventually leaves the orbit by sinking into the floor of the orbit and leaving via the infraorbital foramen. At this stage it becomes known as the infraorbital nerve.

c. False It is the *superior* orbital fissure which lies between the greater and lesser wings of the sphenoid bone. The inferior orbital fissure lies between the orbital surface of the maxilla and the greater wing of the sphenoid.

d. False It transmits the zygomatic branch of the *maxillary* nerve, which is a sensory nerve. The facial nerve also has zygomatic branches. They are motor to the muscles of facial expression in the zygomatic region.

e. False The infraorbital artery is a branch of the maxillary artery. It accompanies the infraorbital nerve.

17. The extraocular muscles include:
   a. The inferior oblique muscle, which is supplied by the trochlear nerve.
   b. The medial rectus, which is supplied by the abducent nerve.
   c. The superior oblique muscle, which pulls the eyeball upwards.
   d. Levator palpebrae superioris, which has both voluntary and involuntary muscle fibres.
   e. Sphincter pupillae, which is innervated by the oculomotor nerve.

18. The trochlear nerve:
   a. Emerges from the dorsal aspect of the midbrain.
   b. Supplies the superior oblique muscle only.
   c. Leaves the anterior cranial fossa through the superior orbital fissure.
   d. Will lead to diplopia when affected unilaterally.

17. a. False The inferior oblique is supplied by the inferior branch of the oculomotor nerve. It is the *superior* oblique which is supplied by the trochlear nerve.

b. False The medial rectus is also supplied by the inferior branch of the oculomotor nerve. It is the *lateral* rectus which is supplied by the abducent nerve. An easy way to remember the innervation of the extraocular muscles is to remember that the trochlear innervates the superior oblique, the abducent innervates the lateral rectus, and the oculomotor innervates all the rest.

c. False Even though it is a difficult concept to imagine, the superior oblique muscle does turn the eye downwards and outwards. This is because it inserts into the posterior half of the eyeball. The inferior oblique will move the eye upwards and outwards.

d. True They are innervated via the oculomotor nerve which carries the motor fibres, both somatic and parasympathetic, in addition to the sympathetic fibres which originate from the spinal cord in the upper thoracic level.

e. False Sphincter pupillae is not an extraocular muscle. It is however innervated by the oculomotor nerve.

18. a. True It is unique in this aspect and a useful criterion in attempting to identify the nerve. All the other cranial nerves exit from the ventral or lateral aspects of the brainstem. It is also the least likely cranial nerve to be preserved in anatomical specimens.

b. True It is therefore a very fine nerve. It has been named trochlear, as the only muscle it supplies passes through a trochlea – the superior oblique muscle.

c. False It does exit via the superior orbital fissure, but this is an aperture between the cavity of the orbit and the *middle* cranial fossa.

d. True Paralysis of the trochlear nerve alone is rare and difficult to detect clinically. The patient would be unable to look down fully, and attempting to look downwards would lead to diplopia.

19. The abducent nerve:
    a. Has a long intracranial course.
    b. Supplies the lateral rectus muscle.
    c. Leaves the skull via the superior orbital fissure.
    d. Carries motor and parasympathetic fibres.

20. The trigeminal nerve:
    a. Has the nerve of the first pharyngeal arch as one of its branches.
    b. Is a purely sensory nerve.
    c. Arises from nuclei in the brainstem and upper spinal cord.
    d. Arises from the ventral aspect of the midbrain.
    e. Has a branch which passes through the superior orbital fissure.

19. a. True It is for this reason that it is commonly affected in non-specific intracranial conditions such as benign intracranial hypertension (pseudotumour cerebri).

    b. True This is the only muscle it supplies.

    c. True Along with the oculomotor, trochlear and ophthalmic branch of the trigeminal nerve (see Head and neck question 15).

    d. False It does not carry any parasympathetic fibres. It only carries motor fibres to the lateral rectus muscle and a few proprioceptive fibres from that muscle.

20. a. True The mandibular nerve is the nerve of the first pharyngeal arch and it is of course the third branch of the trigeminal nerve.

    b. False The mandibular branch of the trigeminal nerve is also motor to the muscles of mastication.

    c. True The motor nuclei are in the pons. The sensory nuclei lie in the midbrain, pons, medulla and cervical cord.

    d. False The trigeminal nerve arises as a motor root and a sensory root from the ventral aspect of the pons laterally, and they converge on the trigeminal ganglion.

    e. True This is the ophthalmic branch of the trigeminal nerve (see Head and neck question 15).

21. The ophthalmic branch of the trigeminal nerve:
   a. Has a branch which is secretomotor to the lacrimal gland.
   b. Has a branch which is sensory to the forehead.
   c. Has a branch which is sensory to the nasal mucosa.
   d. Carries sympathetic and parasympathetic fibres.
   e. Has a branch which passes through the cribriform plate of the ethmoid bone.

22. The maxillary nerve:
   a. Is a purely sensory nerve.
   b. Leaves the skull via the foramen ovale.
   c. Has branches which are sensory to the nasal mucosa.
   d. Carries sensation from all the upper teeth and gums.
   e. Is sensory to the lower eyelid and conjunctiva.

21. a. True   This is the lacrimal branch of the ophthalmic nerve.
    b. True   This is the frontal branch of the ophthalmic nerve. It divides into the supraorbital and supratrochlear nerves, which are sensory to the forehead.
    c. True   This is the nasociliary branch of the ophthalmic nerve.
    d. True   The sympathetic fibres are carried in the long ciliary nerve and the parasympathetic fibres are carried in the short ciliary nerves. Both arise from the nasociliary branch of the ophthalmic nerve.
    e. True   This is the nasociliary nerve, which is called the anterior ethmoidal nerve after it has given off its branches (infratrochlear, posterior ethmoidal and long and short ciliary nerves). As the anterior ethmoidal nerve, it passes briefly to the anterior cranial fossa and exits again through the cribriform plate of the ethmoid bone to become the external nasal nerve.

22. a. True   The only motor fibres carried by the trigeminal nerve are destined for the muscles of mastication and are carried by its mandibular branch.
    b. False   It is the *mandibular* branch of the trigeminal nerve which exits through the foramen ovale. The maxillary nerve leaves the skull through the *foramen rotundum*.
    c. True   The branches of the maxillary nerve which are sensory to the nasal mucosa are the nasopalatine, the posterior superior lateral and medial nasal nerves and the greater palatine nerve.
    d. True   This is through the anterior, middle and posterior superior alveolar nerves.
    e. True   This is via the palpebral branches of the infraorbital nerve. The infraorbital nerve is the continuation of the maxillary nerve. It acquires this new name when it sinks into the floor of the orbit and exits from the infraorbital foramen.

23. The mandibular nerve:
    a.   Supplies the temporalis muscle.
    b.   Is sensory to the temporomandibular joint.
    c.   Has the buccal nerve as one of its branches, which is sensory to the cheek and its mucous membrane and motor to the buccinator muscle.
    d.   Carries sensation and taste from the anterior two-thirds of the tongue via one of its branches.
    e.   Is motor to the mylohyoid muscle and the anterior belly of the digastric.

24. The facial nerve:
    a.   Is the nerve of the third pharyngeal arch.
    b.   Arises from nuclei in the pons and medulla.
    c.   Emerges from the brainstem as a series of rootlets between the pyramid and the olive.
    d.   Leaves the middle cranial fossa through the internal acoustic meatus along with the vestibulocochlear nerve and the nervus intermedius.
    e.   Exits from the skull through the stylomastoid foramen.

23. a. True Temporalis is a muscle of mastication and is therefore supplied by the mandibular nerve.

b. True As the mandibular nerve supplies the muscles which move the temporomandibular joint, it also supplies the joint (Hilton's law).

c. False The buccal nerve is one of the branches of the mandibular nerve but it is a purely sensory nerve. Buccinator is supplied by the buccal branch of the facial nerve.

d. True This is via the lingual nerve. Taste sensation is carried by the chorda tympani which ultimately joins the facial nerve.

e. True The posterior belly is innervated by the facial nerve.

24. a. False The facial nerve is the nerve of the *second* pharyngeal arch. The nerve of the third pharyngeal arch is the glossopharyngeal nerve.

b. True The motor nucleus and the nucleus of the nervus intermedius are in the pons. The sensory nucleus is in the medulla.

c. False The facial nerve emerges from the junction between the pons and the medulla. It is the hypoglossal nerve which emerges as a series of rootlets between the pyramid and the olive.

d. False The facial nerve does pass through the internal acoustic meatus, along with the vestibulocochlear nerve and the nervus intermedius. The internal acoustic meatus, however, lies in the *posterior* cranial fossa.

e. True It leaves the posterior cranial fossa through the internal acoustic meatus, winds its way through the middle ear, and exits from the stylomastoid foramen.

25. The facial nerve:
  a. Supplies the stapedius muscle.
  b. Is sensory to the tympanic membrane.
  c. Is motor to the platysma muscle.
  d. Carries taste sensation from the anterior two-thirds of the tongue.

26. The vestibulocochlear (VIII) nerve:
  a. Emerges from the upper medulla.
  b. Leaves the skull through the jugular foramen.
  c. Arises from nuclei in the pons and medulla.
  d. Is tested prior to diagnosing brain death.
  e. Has a branch which is motor to stapedius.

27. The glossopharyngeal nerve:
  a. Carries taste sensation from the posterior one-third of the tongue.
  b. Is motor to styloglossus.
  c. Is sensory to the hard and soft palate.
  d. Is sensory to the middle ear.
  e. Carries secretomotor fibres to the small salivary glands in the oropharynx.

25. a. True The stapedius muscle is derived from the second
pharyngeal arch and is therefore supplied by the
nerve of that arch – the facial.

   b. True This is via its tympanic branches.

   c. True This is through its cervical branch. The platysma is
a muscle of facial expression and is therefore
supplied by the facial nerve.

   d. True This is via the chorda tympani which travels with
the lingual nerve – a branch of the mandibular
(V_3).

26. a. False It emerges from the groove between the pons and
the medulla.

   b. False It leaves the skull through the internal acoustic
meatus. The cranial nerves which exit through the
jugular foramen are IX, X and XI.

   c. True It arises from two cochlear nuclei in the medulla
and four vestibular nuclei in the pons and medulla.

   d. True As part of the series of tests which are performed
to confirm brain death, ice-cold water is irrigated
into the external auditory canal. Absence of
vestibulo-ocular reflexes indicates brainstem death.

   e. False The vestibulocochlear nerve is a purely sensory
nerve, conveying sound reception and balance only.
Stapedius is supplied by the facial nerve.

27. a. True Taste from the anterior two-thirds of the tongue is
carried by the chorda tympani of the facial nerve.
Its fibres travel with the lingual nerve, a branch of
the mandibular (V_3).

   b. False Styloglossus is one of the muscles of the tongue
and is therefore innervated by the hypoglossal
nerve. Note that there are three muscles arising
from the styloid process, and each one is innervated
by a different cranial nerve. Stylohyoid is
innervated by the facial, stylopharyngeus by the
glossopharyngeal and styloglossus by the
hypoglossal.

   c. False The glossopharyngeal nerve is sensory to the
tongue, pharynx, soft palate and the tonsils. The
hard palate is supplied by the greater palatine
branch of the maxillary nerve (V_2).

   d. True This is via its tympanic branch.

   e. True It is also secretomotor to the parotid gland.

28. The glossopharyngeal nerve:
    a.   Is the nerve of the fourth pharyngeal arch.
    b.   Carries motor, sensory, parasympathetic and taste fibres.
    c.   Exits from the skull via the jugular foramen with the vagus, accessory and hypoglossal nerves.
    d.   Carries special sensory impulses from the carotid sinus and body.
    e.   Arises as a series of rootlets between the medulla and the olive.

29. The vagus nerve:
    a.   Is sensory to a small area of skin in the lower part of the external ear and the external auditory meatus.
    b.   Is motor to the muscles of the soft palate via the pharyngeal plexus.
    c.   Acts with the glossopharyngeal nerve to mediate the gag reflex.
    d.   Innervates the gut down to the transverse colon.

28. a. False It is the nerve of the *third* pharyngeal arch. The
nerve of the fourth pharyngeal arch is the superior
laryngeal branch of the vagus (X).

    b. True It is motor to stylopharyngeus, sensory to the
tongue, palate and pharynx, secretomotor to the
parotid, pharyngeal and lingual glands, and carries
taste from the posterior one-third of the tongue.

    c. False It exits via the jugular foramen along with the
vagus and accessory nerves. The hypoglossal nerve
passes through its own foramen.

    d. True This is via the carotid sinus nerve which carries
sensory input from the baroreceptors of the carotid
sinus and the chemoreceptors of the carotid body.

    e. True It arises in sequence above the rootlets of the
accessory and vagus nerves.

29. a. True This is via its auricular branch, and this may
account for the fainting (vasovagal attack) which
can accompany syringing of the ear. The skin of
the rest of the ear is supplied by the great auricular
and auriculotemporal nerves. The former arises
from C_2 and C_3. The latter is a branch of the
mandibular nerve (V_3).

    b. True The glossopharyngeal nerve also contributes to the
pharyngeal plexus.

    c. True Sensation is mediated via the glossopharyngeal
nerve and there is reflex contraction mediated by
the vagus nerve.

    d. True It is the cranial nerve with the widest distribution.

30. The superior laryngeal nerve:
   a. Is the nerve of the fourth pharyngeal arch.
   b. Is a purely sensory nerve.
   c. Divides into the external and recurrent laryngeal nerves.
   d. Affects the pitch of the voice when damaged.

31. The accessory nerve:
   a. Supplies the skeletal muscles of the pharynx and palate via its cranial component.
   b. Has a spinal component which is sensory to the posterolateral aspect of the neck.
   c. Is motor to sternocleidomastoid.
   d. Has a spinal component which emerges as a series of rootlets from the upper five to six cervical segments of the spinal cord.
   e. Has a cranial component whose fibres arise from the nucleus ambiguus, which lies in the midbrain.

32. The hypoglossal nerve:
   a. Arises as rootlets at a more cranial level than the lowest rootlets of the accessory (XI) nerve.
   b. Is motor to palatoglossus.
   c. Carries fibres from C_{1-3}.
   d. Is motor to the mylohyoid.

30. a. True The nerves of the pharyngeal arches are: mandibular (I), facial (II), glossopharyngeal (III), superior laryngeal (IV) and recurrent laryngeal (VI).

b. False It is motor to cricothyroid and cricopharyngeus via its external laryngeal branch.

c. False It divides into the internal and external laryngeal nerves. The recurrent laryngeal nerve arises from the vagus.

d. True Injury of the external laryngeal branch of the superior laryngeal nerve, e.g. following thyroidectomy, will lead to decreased tension in the vocal cord on the affected side due to weakness or paralysis of the cricothyroid. This will lead to hoarseness or inability to produce high-pitched sounds – a major disability if the patient is an opera singer!

31. a. True These fibres travel with the vagus nerve.

b. False The spinal component of the accessory nerve is purely motor.

c. True The spinal component is motor to sternocleidomastoid and trapezius.

d. True The spinal component emerges from the upper five to six cervical segments of the spinal cord, but it is mainly from C_{2-4}.

e. False The cranial fibres arise from the nucleus ambiguus, which lies in the *medulla*. These fibres supply the musculature derived from the branchial arches.

32. a. True The hypoglossal nerve arises intracranially, whereas the lowest rootlets of the accessory nerve arise from the upper cervical cord.

b. False The hypoglossal nerve is motor to all the intrinsic and extrinsic muscles of the tongue except palatoglossus, which is supplied by the pharyngeal plexus (IX and X).

c. False It carries fibres from C_1 only, which leave the hypoglossal nerve, forming the superior root of the ansa cervicalis. C_2 and C_3 form the inferior root of the ansa cervicalis.

d. False Mylohyoid is supplied by its own nerve, which is a branch of the mandibular nerve (V_3).

33. The recurrent laryngeal nerve:
   a. Supplies the trachea and the oesophagus.
   b. Has a longer course on the right side.
   c. Is the nerve of the sixth pharyngeal arch.
   d. Supplies the posterior cricoarytenoid muscle.
   e. Is sensory to the larynx below the vocal folds.

34. The suprahyoid muscles include:
   a. The digastric muscle which receives its nerve supply from the cervical plexus.
   b. Stylohyoid which elevates the hyoid bone during swallowing.
   c. The digastric muscle, which has an intermediate tendon that is held down by a fibrous sling.
   d. Omohyoid, which is supplied by the ansa cervicalis.
   e. A pair of muscles which form the floor of the mouth.

33. a. True The recurrent laryngeal nerve has cardiac branches, and also supplies the trachea and oesophagus on its way back up to the larynx.

b. False The recurrent laryngeal nerve hooks around the subclavian artery on the right side, whereas the left recurrent laryngeal nerve travels further, as it hooks around the ligamentum arteriosum.

c. True Two of the branches of the vagus are pharyngeal arch nerves. The superior laryngeal is the nerve of the fourth pharyngeal arch, and the recurrent laryngeal nerve is the nerve of the sixth pharyngeal arch (see Head and neck question 30).

d. True The recurrent laryngeal nerve supplies all the intrinsic muscles of the larynx except cricothyroid, which is supplied by the external laryngeal nerve. The posterior cricoarytenoids are the only muscles which open the rima glottidis. Paralysis of both these muscles can have life-threatening consequences.

e. True The recurrent laryngeal nerve is sensory to the mucous membrane of the larynx below the vocal folds; the internal laryngeal nerve supplies the mucous membrane above the vocal folds.

34. a. False It receives its nerve supply from two different cranial nerves – the trigeminal (V) and the facial (VII). Its anterior belly is supplied by the nerve to the mylohyoid, which arises from the mandibular nerve (V_3), whereas the posterior belly is supplied by the facial (VII).

b. True Stylohyoid arises from the styloid process and inserts into the greater horn of the hyoid bone. Its contraction would therefore elevate the hyoid bone and this occurs during swallowing.

c. True This fibrous sling is attached to the lesser horn of the hyoid bone.

d. False The omohyoid muscle is supplied by the ansa cervicalis. It is, however, an *infrahyoid* muscle.

e. True These are the two mylohyoid muscles which arise from the mylohyoid lines on the inner surface of each side of the mandible and unite in the midline in a raphe which extends from the chin to the hyoid bone.

35. The infrahyoid muscles:
a. Are all innervated by the ansa cervicalis except thyrohyoid.
b. Include sternohyoid, which inserts into the outer surface of the medial end of the clavicle.
c. Include omohyoid, which has an anterior and posterior belly.
d. Include a muscle which extends from the oblique line of the thyroid cartilage to the greater horn of the hyoid bone.

36. The thyroid gland:
a. Is made up of two lobes joined by an isthmus which overlies the fifth, sixth and seventh tracheal rings.
b. Is supplied by a branch of the internal carotid artery.
c. Has the recurrent laryngeal nerves running in close proximity to the superior thyroid arteries.
d. Lies deep to the pretracheal fascia.
e. Contains cells which have developed from the fifth pharyngeal pouch.

35. a. True   Thyrohyoid is supplied by C_1 fibres which are carried by the hypoglossal nerve.

    b. False Sternocleidomastoid inserts into the outer surface of the medial end of the clavicle. Sternohyoid inserts into its *inner* surface.

    c. False It is the digastric muscle which has anterior and posterior bellies. The omohyoid has *superior* and *inferior* bellies.

    d. True   This is the thyrohyoid muscle.

36. a. False The isthmus of the thyroid overlies the third, fourth and fifth tracheal rings. This is the recommended site for tracheostomy; the isthmus of the thyroid gland is divided and an opening is made in the second and third tracheal rings.

    b. False The internal carotid artery has no branches in the neck. The *external* carotid artery does supply the thyroid gland via one of its branches – the superior thyroid artery.

    c. False The recurrent laryngeal nerves lie in close proximity to the *inferior* thyroid arteries and may be damaged when ligating the latter. The *external* laryngeal nerves lie in close proximity to the superior thyroid arteries and may also be damaged during thyroid surgery. This will result in an inability to produce high-pitched sounds (see Head and neck question 30).

    d. True   It is for this reason that the thyroid gland moves upwards along with the larynx during swallowing.

    e. True   These are the parafollicular cells which secrete calcitonin. The rest of the thyroid gland develops from an endodermal proliferation in the midline between the junction of the anterior two-thirds and posterior one-third of the tongue, at the point demarcated by the foramen caecum. The thyroid migrates from here caudally to reach its adult position, remaining in communication with its origin via the thyroglossal duct. It is for this reason that thyroid tissue may be found anywhere along this tract.

37. The parathyroid glands:
 a.   Develop from the third and fourth pharyngeal pouches.
 b.   Are fairly constant in position.
 c.   Usually receive their blood supply from branches of the superior thyroid artery.
 d.   Include the inferior parathyroid glands which lie in close proximity to the recurrent laryngeal nerves.
 e.   Include the superior parathyroid glands which usually lie on the posterior aspect of the lateral lobes of the thyroid gland.

38. The submandibular gland:
 a.   Is purely serous.
 b.   Consists of two parts.
 c.   Is crossed by the lingual artery.
 d.   Has its duct opening at the level of the second upper molar tooth.

37. a. True The superior parathyroid glands develop from the fourth pharyngeal pouch, whereas the inferior parathyroid glands, along with the thymus, develop from the third pharyngeal pouch.
    b. False The superior parathyroid glands are fairly constant in position, whereas the inferior parathyroids are notorious for being located in remote sites.
    c. False All four parathyroid glands usually receive their blood supply from branches of the inferior thyroid artery.
    d. True They usually lie between the recurrent laryngeal nerve and the inferior thyroid artery.
    e. True This is usually at the level of the junction of the upper and middle thirds of the lateral lobe of the thyroid gland.

38. a. False It is a mixed mucous and serous salivary gland.
    b. True These are the larger superficial and the smaller deep parts which are separated by the mylohyoid muscle.
    c. False It is crossed by the *facial* artery. The lingual artery lies in a much deeper plane.
    d. False This is the anatomical landmark for the opening of the *parotid* duct. The submandibular duct opens in the floor of the mouth near the frenulum.

39. The internal jugular vein:
a. Emerges from the jugular foramen as the continuation of the straight sinus.
b. Passes through the foramen transversarium in the cervical vertebrae.
c. Has the vagus nerve between it and the internal carotid artery in the upper part of the neck.
d. Receives the superior and middle thyroid veins.

40. Scalenus anterior:
a. Arises from the anterior tubercles of the lower two cervical vertebrae.
b. Inserts on to the first rib.
c. Is innervated by the ansa cervicalis.
d. Has the vagus nerve lying across it, extending from its lateral to its medial border as it passes from above downwards.
e. Separates the subclavian artery from the subclavian vein.

41. The temporalis muscle:
a. Is a muscle of mastication.
b. Inserts into both outer and inner surfaces of the mandible.
c. Lies deep to the masseter muscle.
d. Is supplied by branches of the mandibular nerve (V$_3$).

39. a. False It does emerge from the jugular foramen, but it is the continuation of the *sigmoid* sinus.
   b. False Never! Do not confuse the internal jugular vein with the vertebral vessels.
   c. True They all lie within the loose part of the carotid sheath.
   d. True The inferior thyroid veins drain into the brachiocephalic veins.

40. a. False It arises from the anterior tubercles of C_{3-6}.
   b. True This is at the scalene tubercle which lies on the inner border of the first rib.
   c. False It is innervated segmentally by the anterior rami of C_5 and C_6.
   d. False This is the course of the *phrenic* nerve. The vagus nerve lies medial to scalenus anterior.
   e. True The subclavian vein lies anterior to scalenus anterior; the artery lies posterior to it.

41. a. True Its anterior fibres lift the mandible, whereas its posterior fibres retract it.
   b. True However, its main tendinous insertion is on the inner surface of the mandible.
   c. True Masseter is a fairly superficial muscle which can be easily felt contracting when clenching the jaw.
   d. True The mandibular nerve supplies all the muscles of mastication.

42. The parotid gland:
    a.   Is a mainly mucous salivary gland.
    b.   Lies within the parotid sheath.
    c.   Contains the final bifurcation of the external carotid artery embedded within its glandular tissue.
    d.   Has the retromandibular vein lying between the facial nerve and the external carotid artery.
    e.   Has its duct which runs over the masseter muscle and then pierces buccinator to reach its orifice.

43. The muscles of mastication include:
    a.   The lateral pterygoid muscle, which arises from the infratemporal surface of the skull and the lateral pterygoid plate.
    b.   Masseter, which arises from the zygomatic arch.
    c.   Orbicularis oris, which is innervated by the mandibular nerve.
    d.   The lateral pterygoid muscles, which are powerful grinding muscles which move the mandible from side to side.
    e.   The medial pterygoid, which arises via two heads from the lateral pterygoid plate and the maxilla and palatine bone.

42. a. False   The parotid gland is mainly serous, but it does contain a few scattered mucous elements.

  b. True   The parotid sheath is tough and unyielding. This leads to the pain which occurs during conditions such as mumps (viral parotitis) due to swelling of the gland within its tight sheath.

  c. True   The external carotid artery divides into the superficial temporal and maxillary arteries within the substance of the parotid gland.

  d. True   This is an unusual situation where the nerve lies superficial, the vein is in the middle, and the artery lies deep to it. A similar relationship occurs in the popliteal fossa.

  e. True   The parotid duct can be palpated over the clenched masseter muscle. The parotid duct then pierces the buccinator muscle to reach its opening, which is at the level of the second upper molar tooth.

43. a. True   Its tendon inserts just beneath the mandibular head and into the articular disc of the temporomandibular joint.

  b. True   It inserts on to the ramus of the mandible. Its contraction therefore elevates the mandible and closes the jaws.

  c. False   Orbicularis oris is not a muscle of mastication. It is a muscle of facial expression and it is therefore innervated by the facial nerve, not the mandibular.

  d. False   The lateral pterygoid muscles actively open the jaws when they contract. It is the *medial* pterygoids which move the mandible from side to side, helping to chew the food.

  e. True   Both medial and lateral pterygoid muscles arise from the *lateral* pterygoid plate. The lateral pterygoid muscle arises from its lateral surface and the medial pterygoid muscle arises from its medial surface. The medial pterygoid plate gives attachment to the pharynx. The medial pterygoid muscle arises via two heads – the deep head which arises from the lateral pterygoid plate, and the superficial head which arises from the maxilla and the palatine bone.

44. The branches of the maxillary artery include:
    a.   The middle meningeal artery, which enters the skull through the foramen spinosum.
    b.   The inferior alveolar artery, which supplies the pulps of the teeth in the lower jaw.
    c.   The superficial temporal artery, whose pulsations can be felt in the forehead.
    d.   Branches to the medial and lateral pterygoid muscles and temporalis.

45. The larynx:
    a.   Contains three unpaired cartilaginous structures.
    b.   Contains three paired cartilaginous structures.
    c.   Has the transverse arytenoid muscles posteriorly which are innervated by the recurrent laryngeal nerve.
    d.   Has the posterior cricoarytenoid muscle which opens the vocal cords.
    e.   Is the organ of phonation, and this is its primary function.

44. a. True This is the artery which is implicated in the majority of extradural haematomas following head injuries. There is usually a skull fracture in the temporal region, and the jagged ends of the bone tear the middle meningeal artery, leading to extravasation of arterial blood intracranially. It is often taught (though rarely practised) that when all else fails to control the bleeding from a damaged middle meningeal artery when evacuating an extradural haematoma, the haemorrhage can be controlled by inserting a matchstick into the foramen spinosum!

    b. True It runs in the canal within the mandible.

    c. False The superficial temporal artery is one of the two terminal branches of the external carotid artery, the other being the maxillary artery itself.

    d. True It can therefore be said that the maxillary artery provides the blood supply to the muscles of mastication which are supplied by the mandibular nerve.

45. a. True These are the cricoid and thyroid cartilages and the epiglottis.

    b. True These are the arytenoid, cuneiform and corniculate cartilages.

    c. True All the intrinsic muscles of the larynx are innervated by the recurrent laryngeal nerve except the cricothyroid muscle, which is innervated by the external laryngeal branch of the superior laryngeal nerve.

    d. True The posterior cricoarytenoid also draws the arytenoids downwards.

    e. False The main function of the larynx is protecting the airway during deglutition. Phonation has developed as a secondary function in humans. It also has a function in increasing intra-abdominal pressure during straining and coughing.

46. The nasal cavity:
    a. Contains mucous and serous glands.
    b. Has a floor which is made up of the hard and soft palate.
    c. Contains the superior concha which is the largest of the three conchae.
    d. Contains the opening of the nasolacrimal duct which opens into the inferior meatus.

47. The paranasal air sinuses:
    a. Are lined by simple columnar epithelium interspersed with mucous and serous glands.
    b. Include the maxillary sinus which may have the roots of the upper three molar teeth projecting into it.
    c. All open into the middle meatus except the anterior ethmoidal air cells which open into the superior meatus.
    d. Include the sphenoidal air sinus which receives its blood supply from a branch of the middle cerebral artery.
    e. Include the frontal air sinus which receives its nerve supply from the supraorbital and supratrochlear nerves.

46. a. True The serous secretion humidifies the inspired air, whereas the mucous secretion is said to prevent particulate matter from entering any further into the respiratory passages.

b. False The floor of the nasal cavity is the hard palate. The soft palate separates the nasopharynx from the oropharynx.

c. False It is the inferior concha which is the largest of the three.

d. True The opening of the nasolacrimal duct lies in the anterior part of the inferior meatus just beneath the anterior end of the inferior turbinate.

47. a. False The paranasal air sinuses are lined by respiratory epithelium, i.e. pseudostratified columnar ciliated epithelium with goblet cells.

b. True Sometimes the roots of the upper premolar teeth also project into the maxillary air sinus.

c. False All the paranasal air sinuses open into the middle meatus except the *posterior* ethmoidal air cells which open into the superior meatus and the sphenoid air sinus which opens into the sphenoethmoidal recess, above and behind the superior concha (see Head and neck question 3).

d. False This is absolute nonsense! The blood supply of the sphenoid air sinus is from the maxillary artery via its posterior ethmoidal and sphenopalatine branches.

e. True The supraorbital and supratrochlear nerves are branches of the frontal nerve which arises from the ophthalmic (V_1) nerve. They are sensory to the skin of the forehead, and supply the mucous membrane of the frontal air sinus via branches that pierce the frontal bone.

48. The tongue:
    a. Has the lateral glossoepiglottic fold joining it to the epiglottis.
    b. Is made up entirely of muscle fibres which move it in all directions.
    c. Is connected to the soft palate and the posterior wall of the pharynx by the anterior and posterior pillars of the fauces.
    d. Receives its blood supply from the lingual artery.
    e. Has a lymphatic drainage to the deep cervical lymph nodes of the same side only.

49. The extrinsic muscles of the tongue include:
    a. Genioglossus, the smallest of the extrinsic muscles of the tongue which draws the tongue forward.
    b. Styloglossus, which arises from the styloid process and the stylohyoid ligament.
    c. Hyoglossus, which is innervated by the glossopharyngeal nerve.
    d. Styloglossus, which retracts the tongue.
    e. The mylohyoid muscle, which pulls the tongue downwards.

48. a. False In spite of its name, the lateral glossoepiglottic fold
does not attach to the tongue. It is a mucosal fold
covering a fibrous framework which connects the
epiglottis to the greater horn of the hyoid bone.
   b. False The posterior one-third of the tongue has a large
amount of lymphoid tissue. The whole tongue also
has a large number of serous and mucous glands.
It obviously also has an epithelium with its
specialized papillae. The orientation of its skeletal
muscle fibres does indeed help move it in all
directions.
   c. False The anterior pillar of the fauces (the palatoglossal
arch) joins the posterolateral aspect of the tongue
to the soft palate. The posterior pillar of the fauces
(the palatopharyngeal arch) connects the
oropharynx and the soft palate.
   d. True The lingual artery is, of course, one of the branches
of the external carotid artery.
   e. False The tongue is notorious for the crossing-over which
can occur in its lymphatic drainage, especially from
its posterior part.

49. a. False Genioglossus does draw the tongue forwards,
however, it is the *largest* of all the extrinsic muscles
of the tongue.
   b. True Its fibres pass forwards to be inserted into the side
of the tongue.
   c. False All the intrinsic and extrinsic muscles of the tongue
are supplied by the hypoglossal nerve except
palatoglossus which is supplied by the pharyngeal
plexus.
   d. True Since the attachments of styloglossus are the styloid
process and the side of the tongue, it is obvious
that its contraction would retract the tongue.
   e. False The mylohyoid muscle forms the floor of the
mouth and is *not* an extrinsic muscle of the tongue.

50. The external ear:

a. Receives sensory innervation via the great auricular and lesser occipital nerves which carry fibres from C_3 and C_4.

b. Has intrinsic and extrinsic muscles which are supplied by the facial nerve.

c. Receives its blood supply mainly from a branch of the external carotid artery.

d. Is separated from the middle ear by the tympanic membrane which is supplied on its outer surface by a branch of the mandibular nerve.

e. Also has a sensory supply from both the facial and vagus nerves.

50. a. False The great auricular and lesser occipital nerves do supply the external ear. However, their fibres arise from C$_2$.

  b. True The intrinsic and extrinsic muscles of the external ear are vestigial in humans, but in lower animals they move the external ear and control the size of the auditory meatus.

  c. True This is the posterior auricular artery.

  d. True This is the auriculotemporal branch of the mandibular nerve which supplies the upper part of the auricle and the external auditory meatus, in addition to the outer surface of the tympanic membrane.

  e. True The facial nerve supplies part of the tympanic membrane and the external auditory meatus, whereas the vagus supplies an area of skin near the mastoid process and part of the tympanic membrane and external meatus via its auricular branch. The glossopharyngeal nerve also provides a nerve supply to the tympanic membrane.

51. The middle ear:
- a. Contains the three ossicles which are joined together by means of synovial joints.
- b. Is connected to the nasopharynx by means of the auditory tube which is lined entirely by respiratory epithelium.
- c. Receives its blood supply via branches of both the internal and external carotid arteries.
- d. Contains the tensor tympani muscle which is supplied by a branch of the mandibular nerve.
- e. Contains the stapes which is attached to the tympanic membrane at the umbo.

52. The membranous labyrinth of the inner ear:
- a. Lies within the osseous labyrinth and is surrounded by the perilymph which drains into the CSF.
- b. Contains the duct of the cochlea which is connected to the middle ear by means of the round window.
- c. Contains the medial, lateral and posterior semicircular ducts.
- d. Receives its blood supply via branches of the internal carotid artery.
- e. Contains the saccule and the utricle which lie within the vestibule.

51. a. True The joints between the three ossicles are synovial, and they thus form a bony chain which transmits the sound vibrations from the tympanic membrane to the inner ear.

 b. False The auditory tube is made up of a lateral bony part and a medial cartilaginous part. The cartilaginous part is lined by respiratory epithelium, but the bony part is lined by mucoperiosteum–columnar epithelium with no glands overlying a thin periosteum.

 c. True The main source of blood to the middle ear is through several branches of the external carotid artery – the maxillary, posterior auricular and ascending pharyngeal and their branches. However, it also receives some blood via the caroticotympanic branches of the internal carotid artery which arise from the internal carotid artery as it passes through the carotid canal which lies in the base of the skull.

 d. True It arises from the auditory tube and is attached to the malleus. Its contraction tenses the tympanic membrane, thus providing a dampening effect to minimize the possibility of damage which can be caused by excessively loud noises.

 e. False It is the *handle of the malleus* which is attached to the tympanic membrane at the umbo.

52. a. True The perilymph drains into the CSF through the aqueduct of the cochlea which opens into the subarachnoid space of the posterior cranial fossa.

 b. True It is by this means that the sound vibrations are transmitted from the middle ear to the endolymph within the duct of the cochlea.

 c. False The three semicircular ducts are the *anterior*, posterior and lateral. There is no medial semicircular duct.

 d. False The blood supply of the inner ear *is* from an intracranial source, but it is via the labyrinthine branches of the *basilar* artery. Some blood also reaches the inner ear via the stylomastoid branch of the posterior auricular artery.

 e. True They lie between the cochlea and the semicircular ducts and are considered to be responsible for static balance, whereas the semicircular ducts are responsible for kinetic balance.

53. Levator palpebrae superioris:
  a. Is one of the extrinsic eye muscles.
  b. Arises from the orbital part of the frontal bone.
  c. Has the frontal nerve lying on its superior surface.
  d. Is made up entirely of smooth muscle.
  e. Inserts mainly into the superior tarsal plate.

54. The bony orbit:
  a. Has a lateral wall which is longer than the medial wall.
  b. Has a medial wall which separates the orbital cavity from the nasal cavity and the ethmoidal air cells.
  c. Has the inferior orbital fissure lying between the medial wall and the floor of the orbit.
  d. Has a roof made up of the orbital part of the frontal bone and the lesser wing of the sphenoid.
  e. Communicates with the anterior cranial fossa through the superior orbital fissure.

53. a. False Levator palpebrae superioris, as its name indicates, moves the upper eyelid, not the eyeball.

b. False It arises further posteriorly from the lesser wing of the sphenoid.

c. True This is a prominent structure which is easily recognized when the roof of the orbital cavity is removed. The thick frontal nerve is seen to lie on the superior surface of the uppermost intraorbital muscle – the levator palpebrae superioris. The trochlear nerve also passes medially across the levator palpebrae superioris but it is a much smaller nerve than the frontal.

d. False Opening one's eyes is not usually an involuntary act!

e. True It also inserts into the skin of the upper eyelid and the superior fornix of the conjunctiva.

54. a. False Both medial and lateral walls of the orbit are equal in length.

b. True It is made up of the frontal process of the maxilla, the lacrimal bone, the orbital plate of the ethmoid bone and the body of the sphenoid bone.

c. False The inferior orbital fissure lies between the *lateral* wall and the floor of the orbit.

d. True The orbital part of the frontal bone lies anteriorly and the lesser wing of the sphenoid lies posteriorly. The latter provides only a minor contribution to the roof of the orbit.

e. False The superior orbital fissure is a communication between the orbit and the *middle* cranial fossa.

55. The nerves of the orbit include:
  a. The optic nerve, which passes through the optic foramen accompanied by the ophthalmic artery.
  b. The three branches of the ophthalmic nerve, which are the anterior and posterior ethmoidal nerves and the lacrimal nerve.
  c. The oculomotor nerve, which carries sympathetic fibres to the smooth-muscle component of levator palpebrae superioris and motor fibres to the ciliary ganglion.
  d. Fibres from the zygomatic nerve which are carried by the lacrimal nerve.
  e. The two long ciliary nerves which are motor to the dilator pupillae.

56. The extraocular muscles:
  a. Include the medial, superior and inferior rectus muscles which turn the eye inwards.
  b. Include the lateral rectus and the superior and inferior oblique muscles which turn the eye outwards.
  c. Include the lateral rectus muscle which is supplied by the trochlear nerve.
  d. Include a muscle supplied by the oculomotor nerve which turns the eye upwards and outwards.
  e. Include the superior oblique which, when paralysed, leads to difficulty in reading and going downstairs due to diplopia.

55. a. True The ophthalmic artery also provides the blood
supply of the optic nerve.

    b. False The three branches of the ophthalmic nerve (V_1)
are the lacrimal, frontal and nasociliary nerves. The
posterior ethmoidal is one of the branches of the
nasociliary, whereas the anterior ethmoidal is the
continuation of the nasociliary nerve itself (see
Head and neck question 21).

    c. True The sympathetic fibres are carried in its superior
division, whereas the motor fibres to the ciliary
ganglion are carried by its inferior division.

    d. True These are the secretomotor fibres to the lacrimal
gland. The fibres of the lacrimal nerve itself are
purely sensory, as it is a branch of the ophthalmic
nerve (V_1).

    e. True They carry sympathetic fibres and have been
transported by the nasociliary nerve.

56. a. True It is obvious that the medial rectus muscle turns the
eye inwards, but due to the site of their insertion,
the superior and inferior recti also play a role in
turning the eye inwards. Acting independently, they
would also obviously move the eye upwards or
downwards respectively.

    b. True The lateral rectus muscle obviously turns the eye
outwards. The superior oblique turns the eye
downwards and outwards, whereas the inferior
oblique moves it upwards and outwards.

    c. False The lateral rectus is supplied by the abducent
nerve. The trochlear nerve supplies the superior
oblique.

    d. True This is the inferior oblique muscle. It is supplied by
the inferior branch of the oculomotor nerve and it
turns the eye upwards and outwards.

    e. True The superior oblique muscle turns the eye outwards
and downwards – a position essential for reading,
going downstairs, and other actions which require
looking downwards, such as sewing and knitting.

57. The falx cerebri:
    a.   Is a fold of dura mater which separates the cerebral hemispheres from the cerebellum.
    b.   Contains the inferior sagittal sinus running within its lower border just above the corpus callosum.
    c.   Contains the superior sagittal sinus which usually drains into the right transverse sinus.
    d.   Contains the straight sinus which lies at its junction with the tentorium cerebelli.
    e.   Is sickle-shaped.

58. The anterior cranial fossa:
    a.   Has part of its floor forming the roof of both orbits.
    b.   Contains the frontal lobes which have the olfactory bulbs lying on their inferior surface.
    c.   Has the foramen caecum which lies immediately posterior to the crista galli in the midline.
    d.   Contains the anterior attachment of the falx cerebri.
    e.   When fractured, may lead to CSF rhinorrhoea if the dura has been breached.

57. a. False Of course not! The falx separates the two cerebral hemispheres. It is the tentorium cerebelli which separates the cerebral hemispheres from the cerebellum. The falx cerebelli partially separates the two cerebellar hemispheres.

   b. True This is one of the ways of approaching the corpus callosum surgically for some forms of intractable epilepsy.

   c. True This is at the level of the internal occipital protuberance.

   d. True The straight sinus drains the inferior sagittal sinus and the great cerebral vein (of Galen). It usually drains into the left transverse sinus.

   e. True Falx is Latin for sickle.

58. a. True This is formed by the orbital plate of the frontal bone.

   b. True The olfactory filaments which pass through the cribriform plate of the ethmoid bone terminate in these olfactory bulbs.

   c. False The foramen caecum lies immediately *anterior* to the crista galli.

   d. True The falx cerebri is attached anteriorly to the crista galli which lies within the anterior cranial fossa.

   e. True Since the anterior cranial fossa also forms the roof of the nasal cavity, any CSF escaping from a breach in the dura would run down through the fracture in the anterior cranial fossa into the patient's nose.

59. The middle cranial fossa:
  a. Contains the pituitary gland which lies just above the sphenoid air sinus.
  b. Contains the optic chiasm which lies immediately anterior to the pituitary gland.
  c. Contains the internal carotid artery which emerges from within the cavernous sinus.
  d. Contains the optic nerve which passes through the cavernous sinus to reach the orbital cavity.

60. The posterior cranial fossa:
  a. Contains the two vertebral arteries which enter through the foramen magnum.
  b. Contains the facial nerve which leaves through the jugular foramen.
  c. Has a wide groove on both sides caused by the right and left transverse venous sinuses.
  d. Has part of its floor formed by the clivus of the occipital bone.
  e. Has the internal occipital crest in the midline which provides attachment to the falx cerebelli.

59. a. True One of the surgical routes to approach the pituitary gland is trans-sphenoidally.

b. False The optic chiasm lies immediately *posterior* to the pituitary gland. A pituitary tumour would compress the optic chiasm leading to a visual field defect (loss of temporal field vision bilaterally – homonymous hemianopia).

c. True The internal carotid artery passes through the carotid canal in the base of the skull to reach the middle cranial fossa where it comes to lie within the cavernous sinus. It gives off the ophthalmic artery when it emerges from the cavernous sinus and subsequently divides into its two terminal branches – the anterior and middle cerebral arteries.

d. False Nonsense! The abducent nerve lies within the cavity of the cavernous sinus, whereas the oculomotor, trochlear, ophthalmic and maxillary nerves lie within its lateral wall. The optic nerve passes medial to it to enter the optic foramen.

60. a. True They arise from the first part of the subclavian artery, pass upwards through the foramina transversaria of the sixth to the second cervical vertebrae, then loop around the transverse process of the atlas and pass through its foramen before piercing the atlanto-occipital membrane and entering the skull through the foramen magnum.

b. False The facial nerve exits through the internal acoustic meatus. It is the glossopharyngeal, vagus and accessory nerves which exit through the jugular foramen.

c. True The right transverse sinus is usually larger than the left, and therefore causes a large indentation on the inner surface of the posterior cranial fossa.

d. True The clivus extends from the foramen magnum to the dorsum sellae.

e. True The falx cerebelli is a small fold of dura which contains the small occipital sinus and protrudes into the shallow indentation between the two cerebellar hemispheres. It is attached to the internal occipital protuberance, the internal occipital crest and the posterior rim of the foramen magnum.

61. In the adult human skull:
   a. The metopic suture separates the two frontal bones.
   b. The bregma is an area on the lateral surface of the skull where there is an H-shaped arrangement of sutures between the frontal, parietal, temporal and sphenoid bones.
   c. The lambdoid suture separates the two parietal bones from the two occipital bones.
   d. The temporal bone contributes to the zygomatic arch.
   e. The superior nuchal line joins the two mastoid processes to the external occipital protuberance.

61. a. False There is only one frontal bone in the adult human skull. The metopic suture is the site of fusion of the two halves of the frontal bone. It is more evident when the two halves of the frontal bone have failed to fuse completely.

b. False The bregma lies on the top of the skull in the midline, between the frontal and two parietal bones, at the site of the anterior fontanelle. The *pterion* is the area surrounding the H-shaped arrangement of sutures on the lateral aspect of the skull. It is clinically significant as the bones are thin in this area and therefore more liable to fracture following trauma. This may subsequently lead to intracranial haemorrhage, and therefore the pterion is the recommended site for the first exploratory burr hole when not guided by computed tomography (CT) scan.

c. False Again, note that there is only one occipital bone in the human skull.

d. True The temporal bone has four parts: petrous (which includes the mastoid process), squamous, tympanic and the styloid process. The zygomatic process of the temporal bone arises from its squamous part.

e. True The superior nuchal line gives origin to the trapezius, sternocleidomastoid and some of the postvertebral muscles.

62. In the cervical spine:
   a.   The posterior longitudinal ligament lies anterior to the spinal cord.
   b.   The vertebral body is about twice the size of the vertebral canal.
   c.   The seventh cervical vertebra has a large prominent bifid spinous process.
   d.   The sixth cervical vertebra carries the carotid tubercle on its body.
   e.   There is a foramen in the transverse process of all the cervical vertebrae.

62. a. True   The anterior and posterior longitudinal ligaments
are named according to their relation to the bodies
of the vertebrae. They therefore both lie anterior to
the spinal cord.

   b. False   In the cervical spine, the vertebral body and the
vertebral canal are of approximately equal size.
This reflects the relatively small size of the vertebral
bodies and large size of the spinal cord at this level.

   c. False   The seventh cervical vertebra does have a large
prominent spinous process and is therefore known
as the vertebra prominens. Its spinous process,
however, differs from that of the other cervical
vertebrae in that it is not bifid.

   d. False   The carotid tubercle lies on the *transverse process*
of the sixth cervical vertebra. It is called the carotid
tubercle because the common carotid artery can be
compressed against it. This can lead to
unconsciousness – a feat much more easily achieved
in old Hollywood movies than in reality!

   e. True   The largest is the foramen in the transverse process
of the atlas vertebra. This is the route taken by the
vertebral arteries running upwards to supply the
brainstem and cerebellum. Note that the foramen
transversarium of the seventh cervical vertebra
transmits the vertebral vein only, as the vertebral
arteries enter through the foramen of the *sixth*
cervical vertebra and proceed upwards.

Histology

1. **With regard to the heart:**
   a. The endothelium sits on a fenestrated basement membrane.
   b. Cardiac myocytes anastomose to form a network.
   c. Chordae tendinae are composed of loose connective tissue.
   d. Visceral serous pericardium is the same as epicardium.
   e. The elements of the conducting system are modified neurons.

2. **In the respiratory tract:**
   a. The upper surface of the epiglottis is lined by respiratory epithelium.
   b. The muscular vocal folds are covered by keratinized stratified squamous epithelium.
   c. Type 1 pneumocytes secrete surfactant.
   d. The nasal cavity is not lined by respiratory epithelium.
   e. There are no mucous glands in bronchioles.

1. a. False The basement membrane is not fenestrated.
   b. False Cardiac myocytes form junctions with each other, consisting of desmosomes, tight junctions and gap junctions. This facilitates the structural integrity of the myocardium, as well as providing a means by which electrical impulses can spread across it. The junctional complexes are the intercalated discs.
   c. False Chordae tendinae have a centre of dense connective tissue, covered by thin endocardium.
   d. True The epicardium is a serous membrane which sometimes can be quite fat-laden. It is in this layer that the coronary vessels may be found.
   e. False The conducting system is composed of modified cardiac myocytes. In histological section they appear large and are often aggregated in bundles, lying between the normal myocytes.

2. a. False The upper surface of the epiglottis is lined by stratified squamous epithelium, which is protective since this surface will come into contact with food, and therefore will be subject to abrasion. Respiratory epithelium (pseudostratified ciliated columnar epithelium with goblet cells) is found on the lower surface.
   b. False The vocal folds are covered by non-keratinized stratified squamous epithelium.
   c. False Type 2 pneumocytes secrete surfactant. Type 1 pneumocytes form the alveolar wall.
   d. False The nasal cavity is nearly all lined by respiratory epithelium, except for the vestibule, where the skin of the external nose loses its keratinized character. Where the nasal epithelium covers the turbinate bones it is continuous with the periosteum, and is referred to as a mucoperiosteum.
   e. True The lining epithelium is much thinner here and acquires a low cuboidal character. All glandular secretions arise from glands situated in the bronchi and trachea.

3. In the alimentary canal:
  a. Mucous neck cells secrete hydrochloric acid.
  b. Chromaffin cells are only found in the suprarenal medulla.
  c. Paneth cells contain muramidase (lysozyme) and immunoglobulin A.
  d. Peyer's patches are more numerous in the ileum.
  e. Taenia coli are a form of parasite which inhabit the large intestine.

3. a. False Hydrochloric acid is secreted by parietal (oxyntic) cells. Mucous neck cells are found close to the surface of the gastric glands and they secrete mucus, not hydrochloric acid.

b. False The chromaffin cells, formerly called argentaffin cells, are part of the APUD system (acronym for **A**mine **P**recursor **U**ptake, **D**ecarboxylase-containing cells), and are derived from the neural crest. They are found scattered throughout the gastrointestinal tract, and in other systems too. They form part of the diffuse neuroendocrine system and are responsible for the local secretion of hormones.

c. True Lying at the bottom of the crypts, these cells contain granules which are characteristically eosinophilic. They also contain dipeptidases and zinc.

d. True Peyer's patches constitute part of the gut-associated lymphoid system and represent unencapsulated lymphoid tissue. This is part of the mucosal immune system, in which immunoglobulin A is a predominant antibody formed to protect the mucosa of the gut.

e. False Taenia coli are the three longitudinal bands of smooth muscle, forming part of the muscularis externa in the large intestine. They are clearly visible with the naked eye. *Taenia saginata* and *T. solium* are the beef and pork tapeworms which are the intestinal parasites.

4. **In the liver:**
   a. Kupffer cells line the canaliculi.
   b. A portal triad consists of branches of the hepatic artery and bile duct, and tributaries of the hepatic vein.
   c. The parenchymal cells of the liver are not in direct contact with blood cells.
   d. The parenchymal cells of the liver are rich in glycogen.
   e. Haemopoiesis occurs in the fetus.

5. **In the urinary system:**
   a. The glomerulus consists of Bowman's capsule, and the afferent and efferent arteriole.
   b. The renal corpuscle consists of Bowman's capsule, the glomerulus and the juxtaglomerular apparatus.
   c. The glomerular space is an artefact.
   d. The proximal convoluted tubules are characterized by numerous infoldings of the basement membrane, as well as numerous mitochondria.
   e. The urinary bladder is lined by stratified non-keratinized squamous epithelium.

4. a. False Kupffer cells line the sinusoids and are phagocytic. They remove effete erythrocytes, and other waste material. In contrast to what was stated in older textbooks they are derived from blood monocytes, and not the septum transversum.

b. False The portal triad or tract consists of a hepatic artery, a hepatic portal vein and a bile duct, *not* a hepatic vein. The bile duct is easily distinguished because it is lined by cuboidal epithelium. The blood vessels are of typical histology, and more than one profile of each of the three structures may be found in a typical transverse section through a portal triad. The hepatic vein is fed by the central vein of a portal lobule, lying, as its name suggests, at the centre of the portal lobule.

c. True The lumen of the sinusoids is incompletely bounded by the cytoplasm of the reticuloendothelial and Kupffer cells. Beneath this is the narrow space of Disse which thus separates the hepatocytes from the deep margin of the reticuloendothelial cells. Since the sinusoidal cells form an incomplete boundary, blood plasma is in direct contact with the hepatocytes, but the hepatocytes are not in contact with the blood cells.

d. True There are a large number of substances stored by hepatocytes. Glycogen can be mobilized from the liver to raise blood glucose levels, and vice versa.

e. True A variety of haemopoietic cells can be found in the fetal liver.

5. a. False The glomerulus consists of just a tuft of capillaries.

b. True The juxtaglomerulus apparatus is a modification of the part of the afferent arteriole as it enters the corpuscle.

c. True It is seen in paraffin sections, but not in frozen sections.

d. False This description fits distal convoluted tubules. The presence of numerous mitochondria reflects the energy-dependent reabsorption processes taking place in the distal tubules. Proximal convoluted tubules are characterized by a microvillous luminal border.

e. False The urinary bladder is lined by transitional epithelium.

6. In the genital system:
   a. The vaginal epithelium is characterized by its most superficial cells being pale and empty, because they are dead.
   b. The ductus deferens is lined by three layers of differently oriented smooth muscle.
   c. The prostate is rich in acid phosphatase and acquires concretions in old age.
   d. An atretic follicle is the result of the regression of a Graafian follicle before ovulation occurs.
   e. The uterine tube is lined by ciliated columnar epithelium.

7. In the digestive system:
   a. The tongue has keratinized epithelium covering its circumvallate papillae.
   b. The tongue has three layers of smooth muscle, each at different orientations.
   c. The serous cells of the parotid gland stain intensely with eosin.
   d. The glycogen in liver cells can be demonstrated with the periodic acid–Schiff method.
   e. There is no submucosa in the gall bladder.

6. a. False The superficial cells of the vaginal epithelium are living cells. Their characteristic appearance is due to the fact that these cells were rich in glycogen which, in paraffin sections, has been dissolved out by the processing method.

   b. True There is an inner longitudinal, middle circular and outer longitudinal smooth-muscle layer.

   c. True The concretions can become so large as to block the glandular ducts, and contribute to the impairment of urine flow through the prostatic urethra, as seen in generalized prostatic hypertrophy. A raised serum acid phosphatase is suggestive of prostatic malignancy.

   d. True These structures are composed of dense connective tissue, and are not to be confused with corpora albicantes, the result of the regression of corpora lutea which are also composed of dense connective tissue.

   e. True The cilia are one of the means by which the ovum and spermatozoa are transported along the length of the tube.

7. a. False The tongue has *non-keratinized* epithelium covering its circumvallate papillae, as well as its fungiform and filiform papillae.

   b. False The tongue has three planes of *skeletal* muscle, each at right angles to one another.

   c. False The serous cells of the parotid gland stain with haematoxylin because they contain material which is acidic, particularly proteins. Eosin stains *basic* material like the granules of eosinophils!

   d. True To confirm the presence of glycogen, the sections should be digested with diastase (saliva is a good source, which is why histochemists may sometimes be seen spitting over the sink on to their slides!) and the periodic acid–Schiff method reapplied. The section should be unreactive.

   e. True There is no submucosa in the gall bladder! The wall of the gall bladder is composed of an epithelium and a muscularis covered either by an adventitia or a serosa.

8. **In the skin:**
   a. The prickle-cell layer can be found in the dermis.
   b. Sweat glands open on to the surface of the skin via spiral channels in the epidermis.
   c. Merkel cells are the antigen-presenting cells.
   d. The hypodermis is regarded as part of the skin.
   e. Arrectores pilorum muscles are skeletal muscle tissue.

9. **In the development of blood cells:**
   a. Megakaryocytes give rise to red blood cells.
   b. Reticulocytes can sometimes be found in peripheral blood.
   c. Plasma cells are found in peripheral blood.
   d. Haematopoiesis in adults takes place in the liver and spleen, as well as the bone marrow.
   e. Production of lymphoid cells takes place in the bone marrow, and to some extent in lymphoid organs.

8. a. False It is found in the epidermis where it forms the thickest layer. The term prickles arises from the appearance of the cells in section. The prickles result from the cell junctions between adjacent squamous epithelial cells.

b. True Sweat glands do indeed open on to the surface of the skin via spiral channels in the epidermis, which are often mistaken for imperfections or artefacts in the epidermis by the novice histologist.

c. False It is the Langerhans cell which is the antigen-presenting cell in skin. Merkel cells are sensory receptors concerned with touch.

d. False The hypodermis is not part of the skin – it is part of the superficial fascia, and in obese individuals may be very substantial.

e. False The arrectores pilorum muscles are smooth-muscle tissue. Their contraction is involuntary, and they are supplied by the sympathetic nervous system.

9. a. False Megakaryocytes give rise to blood platelets or thrombocytes by a process whereby the platelets break off from the cytoplasm of the megakaryocyte.

b. True Reticulocytes can sometimes be found in peripheral blood, but only in circumstances where there is a need for rapid production of red blood cells, i.e. anaemia.

c. False Plasma cells are not normally found in peripheral blood. If they are, then the patient needs to see a consultant haematologist urgently!

d. False Haematopoiesis only occurs in the liver and spleen during fetal life.

e. False It is the other way round. The production of lymphoid cells takes place in the lymphoid organs and to some extent in the bone marrow.

10. In lymphoid organs:
   a. Plasma cells are found in the subcapsular sinuses of lymph nodes.
   b. The periarteriolar lymphatic sheaths are composed mainly of reticulin fibres.
   c. Hassall's corpuscles are found in the cortex of the thymus.
   d. Tonsils are characterized by the crypts of Lieberkühn.
   e. The spleen is characterized by trabeculae which are mainly composed of collagen and elastin.

10. a. True   Plasma cells can be found in the subcapsular sinuses of lymph nodes, though they are most readily identified in the medullary cords.

     b. False   The periarteriolar lymphatic sheaths are composed of T lymphocytes.

     c. False   Hassall's corpuscles are found in the medulla of the thymus. Hassall's corpuscles are epithelial-derived cells from the third pharyngeal pouch in the embryo. They are highly conspicuous in sections of thymus, and are often presented to students in histology examinations.

     d. False   This is nonsense! Crypts are features of tonsils, and it is in them that material can become lodged and infected in tonsillitis, but the crypts of Lieberkühn are to be found in the small intestine.

     e. True   In some animals, though not in humans, there is also smooth muscle, enabling the spleen to contract like a sponge to extrude its stored blood in times of demand, e.g. after haemorrhage.

Neuroanatomy

1. **With regard to the developing brain:**
    a.   The telencephalon gives rise to the cerebral cortex and basal ganglia.
    b.   The diencephalon gives rise to the thalamus.
    c.   The metencephalon gives rise to the pineal gland.
    d.   The myelencephalon gives rise to the pons and midbrain.
    e.   The neurectoderm gives rise to all the autonomic ganglia.

2. **The neurons of the central nervous system:**
    a.   Are associated with three types of glial cells, all derived from ectoderm.
    b.   Are arranged in six layers in the cerebral cortex.
    c.   Differ from those of the peripheral nervous system as regards their myelination.
    d.   Are characterized by synaptic vesicles containing Nissl substance.
    e.   Have axons which are no more than 10 cm in length.

1. a. True   The cerebral cortex and basal ganglia do arise from the telencephalon, the latter arising with the diencephalon from the prosencephalon.
   b. True   The diencephalon gives rise to the thalamus, hypothalamus, pineal gland and the posterior pituitary gland.
   c. False The metencephalon gives rise to the cerebellum and pons.
   d. False The myelencephalon gives rise to the medulla oblongata.
   e. True   The autonomic ganglia are derived from the neural crest, which is derived from neurectoderm.

2. a. False Astrocytes and oligodendrocytes are derived from neurectoderm, but microglial cells are mesoderm-derived.
   b. True   The cerebral cortex has its full complement of six layers by the 18th week of gestation.
   c. True   The neurons of the central nervous system are myelinated by oligodendrocytes, whilst those of the peripheral nervous system are myelinated by Schwann cells.
   d. False Synaptic vesicles contain neurotransmitter substance, e.g. noradrenaline, acetylcholine, whereas Nissl substance is ribonucleic acid of rough endoplasmic reticulum in the cytoplasm of the cell body of the neuron.
   e. False Some axons, notably motor and sensory axons in the somatic nervous system, can be anything up to about 120 cm in length.

3. **The main motor pathway in the central nervous system:**
   a. Is the so-called pyramidal pathway.
   b. Passes through the cerebral peduncles.
   c. Is directed to the intrafusal muscle fibres.
   d. Arises in the premotor cortex of the cerebrum.
   e. Terminates on the ventral horn of the spinal cord.

3. a. True   The pathway consists of two parts – the lateral corticospinal tract, constituting about 85% of the pyramidal pathway, and the anterior corticospinal tract (the other 15%). The former decussates in the pyramids of the medulla, whilst the latter, innervating mainly head, neck and trunk musculature, decussates in the spinal cord, at the level of exit.

b. True   The cerebral peduncles are the main entry and exit point for the principal motor and sensory pathways of the brain.

c. True   Gamma motor neurons control the length and tension of the neuromuscular spindles. Their pattern of firing determines the thresholds of the sensory nerve endings in the spindles, the receptors for the spinal reflex arcs.

d. False   The corticospinal pathway arises in the *motor* cortex, in the parietal lobe of the cerebrum, in the *precentral* gyrus.

e. True   Besides the motor pathway, sensory information and other descending pathways also terminate on the ventral horn neurons, establishing the reflex arc, and thus the ventral horn neuron is often called the final common pathway.

4. The cerebrum:
   a.   Contains the caudate nuclei.
   b.   Contains the dentate nuclei.
   c.   Contains the gracile and cuneate nuclei.
   d.   Contains the lentiform nuclei.
   e.   Contains the thalamic nuclei.

4. a. True The caudate nuclei are paired structures which curve around the thalamus and lentiform nucleus. Each caudate nucleus has a head, body and tail, and lies in contact with the amygdaloid body. They are part of the corpus striatum which modulates the control mechanisms for voluntary movement.

b. False The dentate nucleus is one of the deep nuclei of the cerebellum.

c. False The gracile and cuneate nuclei lie in the medulla. They receive the fibres of the dorsal column (medial lemniscus) pathway which convey information about proprioception, discriminatory touch and vibration.

d. True The lentiform nuclei are part of the corpus striatum, and consist of the globus pallidus and the putamen. Along with the caudate nuclei they are concerned with the control mechanisms for voluntary movement. Disorders of the neural circuits involving the corpus striatum lead to dyskinesias such as Huntington's chorea or Parkinson's disease.

e. True Bordering the third ventricle, the thalamus comprises about four-fifths of the total volume of the diencephalon (thalamus and hypothalamus), and it takes the form of about a dozen nuclei with a variety of motor and sensory cortical and spinal connections. It is the site of relay for the somatosensory pathways *en route* for the sensory cortex, and it sends projections to the motor cortex, and to the auditory and visual cortices.

5. With regard to the blood supply of the brain:
   a. Blockage in the anterior cerebral artery could result in deficits in movement of the leg.
   b. The striate artery, frequently a site of cerebrovascular accidents, is a branch of the posterior cerebral artery.
   c. The posterior cerebral artery supplies the major part of the parietal lobe.
   d. No artery supplying the cerebellum is a direct branch of any of the cerebral arteries.
   e. The pontine arteries supply only the pons.

5. a. True   The motor cortex is located in the precentral gyrus of the frontal lobe. It continues from the lateral to the medial surface of the cerebrum. The blood supply of the motor cortex is from two sources. The middle cerebral artery supplies the major part of that part lying on the lateral surface, whilst the anterior cerebral artery supplies that part lying on the medial surface. The cortical representation of motor function, often referred to as the motor homunculus, is arranged with neurons projecting to feet in the medial part of the gyrus, and those to the head region on the inferolateral part of the gyrus.

  b. False   Though they are often the site of lesions in stroke victims, they are branches of the *middle* cerebral artery.

  c. False   The posterior cerebral artery supplies mainly the occipital lobe, hence its occlusion results in impairments of sight. It also supplies part of the temporal lobe. Most of the parietal lobe is supplied by the middle cerebral artery.

  d. True   There are three arteries supplying the cerebellum: the superior cerebellar artery, arising from the basilar artery, and supplying the cortex, medullary centre and central nuclei. Proximal branches of this vessel supply the pons, superior cerebellar peduncle and the inferior colliculus of the midbrain. The anterior inferior cerebellar artery arises at the convergence of the vertebral arteries as they form the basilar artery and supplies the cortex and deep nuclei and gives rise to small branches to parts of the medulla and pons. The posterior inferior cerebellar arteries, which are branches of the basilar artery, are distributed to the posterior parts of the cerebellum, and its underlying deep nuclei, as well as the medulla.

  e. True   The slender vessels which supply the pons arise from the basilar artery and enter the pons on its ventral surface. Immediately posterior is the labyrinthine artery (sometimes the latter vessel arises from the anterior inferior cerebellar artery), which passes into the inner ear via the internal acoustic meatus to supply the membranous labyrinth (see Head and neck question 52).

6. With regard to the cerebellum:
   a. The flocculonodular lobe represents the larger of the three cerebellar lobes.
   b. The neocerebellum is responsible for equilibrium.
   c. The cortex lies outside the white matter.
   d. Its largest cell type is the so-called Purkinje cell.
   e. Unlike the cerebral cortex, there are only three cortical layers.

7. In the cerebral cortex:
   a. The visual association area in the occipital cortex is much larger than the cortex of the primary visual cortex.
   b. Wernicke's area in the temporal lobe is concerned with the expression of speech.
   c. The auditory centre is located in the superior temporal gyrus.
   d. The prefrontal cortex is categorized as an association cortex.
   e. Olfaction is associated with the insula cortex.

6. a. False The flocculonodular lobe is the smallest lobe of the cerebellum, the posterior lobe being the largest. The third cerebellar lobe is the anterior cerebellar lobe.

b. False The neocerebellum, the newest part of the cerebellum phylogenetically, is formed by the posterior lobe, otherwise known as the pontocerebellum, and is concerned with the regulation of skilled movements.

c. True This applies to both the cerebellum and the cerebrum.

d. True The principal projection of the Purkinje cells is to the deep nuclei of the cerebellum, i.e. the dentate, fastigial, globose and embeliform nuclei.

e. True In the cerebellar cortex there are only three layers (unlike the six in the cerebrum). The smallest of the three is the Purkinje cell layer, characterized by the single row of large Purkinje (multipolar) neurons. Superficial to these neurons is the molecular layer, largely a synaptic layer. Deep to the Purkinje cell layer is the granule cell layer, largely small interneurons. Interspersed amongst these cells are the climbing fibres and the mossy fibres.

7. a. True The visual association cortex relates present to past visual experience and helps in recognition and in appreciation of significance.

b. False It is Broca's area in the inferior frontal gyrus that is responsible for expression. Wernicke's area is concerned with recognition of language: the receptive language centre.

c. True Only the posteromedial part of this gyrus is the primary auditory cortex.

d. True Its main functions are in behaviour monitoring; plans and intentions are evolved here; judgement and foresight are also important roles for this area of the cortex. It therefore has extensive connections with many other parts of the cerebral cortex to acquire information from other senses.

e. True In addition, some of the olfactory projections end in the entorhinal cortex in the temporal lobe, which is part of the limbic system.

8. The sensory pathways of the nervous system include:
 a. The posterior column pathway, whose second-order neurons synapse in the ipsilateral pons.
 b. The lateral spinothalamic tract, which carries proprioceptive information.
 c. The anterior spinothalamic tract, which crosses over at its point of entry.
 d. The spinocerebellar pathways, which only project to the ipsilateral cerebellum.
 e. The spinocerebellar pathways, which gain access to the cerebellum via the middle cerebellar peduncle.

9. The brainstem:
 a. Gives rise to the XIIth cranial nerve between the olive and the pyramid of the pons.
 b. Contains the pontine nuclei which project to the cerebral cortex.
 c. Contains the substantia nigra in the pons.
 d. Has as its only visible part in the midbrain the cerebral peduncles.
 e. Gives rise to the Vth cranial nerve at the pontomedullary junction.

8. a. False The posterior column pathway (sometimes called the medial lemniscus pathway) contains second-order neurons which synapse in the ipsilateral medulla in the cuneate or gracile nuclei. The nerve fibres, whose cell bodies are located in the dorsal root ganglia, pass cranially via the fasciculi cuneatus or gracilis to the appropriate nucleus. From here, after synapsing they pass to the thalamus and as third-order neurons projecting to the somatosensory cortex.

b. False The lateral spinothalamic tract carries information regarding pain and temperature. The anterior spinothalamic pathway mediates fine touch and pressure sensation.

c. True The anterior spinothalamic tract does cross over at its point of entry, as does the lateral spinothalamic tract. The posterior column pathways do not cross over until they reach the medulla.

d. False The dorsal spinocerebellar pathways project only to the ipsilateral cerebellum, whereas the ventral pathway projects to both contralateral and ipsilateral cerebellum.

e. False The anterior and posterior spinocerebellar pathways gain access to the cerebellum via the superior and inferior cerebellar peduncles respectively, and pass to the anterior lobe of the cerebellum.

9. a. False The XIIth cranial nerve does indeed emerge from between the olive and the pyramid, but of the medulla.

b. False The pontine nuclei project to the cerebellum and are concerned with control of fine-skilled movements, relaying information from the motor cortex of the cerebrum to the cerebellum via the middle cerebellar peduncle.

c. False It is the midbrain that contains the substantia nigra. This pigment is lost in the hypokinetic disorder, Parkinson's disease.

d. True These connect the internal capsule with the motor and somatosensory cortices.

e. False The Vth (trigeminal) cranial nerve emerges from the pons. The VIth (abducens), VIIth (facial) and VIIIth (vestibulocochlear) cranial nerves (in addition to the nervus intermedius) arise from the pontomedullary junction.

10. In the cerebral cortex:
   a.   The globus pallidus is part of the lentiform nucleus.
   b.   The claustrum is wholly grey matter.
   c.   The basal ganglia include the vermis.
   d.   The septum pellucidum divides the lateral ventricles.
   e.   The putamen is derived from the diencephalon.

10. a. True The globus pallidus is part of the lentiform nucleus
which itself forms part of the corpus striatum with
the putamen. These are also components of the
basal ganglia and are concerned with motor
control.

 b. True It lies as a thin layer of grey matter just superficial
to the external capsule.

 c. False The vermis is in the midline of the cerebellum.

 d. False The septum pellucidum only separates the anterior
horns of the ventricles.

 e. False The diencephalon gives rise to the thalamus and the
hypothalamus. The putamen is derived from the
telencephalon.

Embryology

1. **The developing heart:**
   a. Arises from the intraembryonic coelom.
   b. Forms in much the same way as a blood vessel.
   c. Is initially a caudal relation of the septum transversum.
   d. Is the first organ to become functional.
   e. Has initially only a single artery and vein arising from it.

1. a. False The developing heart arises from the cardiogenic mesoderm. It develops within the future pericardial cavity, which is part of the intraembryonic coelom.

b. True It is often said that the heart is nothing more than a modified blood vessel, possessing three similar layers. The major difference is in the thickness of its wall and its possession of partitions.

c. True The unsegmented mesoderm from which the heart arises lies immediately caudal to the unsegmented mesoderm of the septum transversum in an unfolded embryo.

d. True During the fourth week the heart becomes functional. This provides a means for further development in the embryo.

e. True Early in subsequent development the arterial end splits into two, the future truncus arteriosus becoming the ascending aorta and the pulmonary trunk. The venous end (the sinus venosus) divides into six, giving rise to the two venae cavae and the four pulmonary veins.

2. **The endoderm of the gut tube gives rise to the parenchyma of the:**
   a. Kidney.
   b. Liver.
   c. Pancreas.
   d. Spleen.
   e. Suprarenal gland.

2. a. False The intermediate mesoderm gives rise to the tubules of the kidney.

   b. True The hepatocytes do arise from the endoderm germ layer. The Kupffer cells, which are not parenchymal cells, are derived from the bone marrow, which is mesodermal in origin. Some older textbooks erroneously state that the Kupffer cells originate from the septum transversum.

   c. True The exocrine and endocrine portions of the pancreas are both derived from endoderm. The pancreas develops as two separate buds, a larger dorsal bud and a smaller ventral bud. The duct systems of the two normally merge and open into the duodenum at the major duodenal papilla, though not uncommonly the duct of the smaller ventral bud persists and opens separately at the minor duodenal papilla.

   d. False Although the spleen develops in the dorsal mesogastrium, it arises from bone-marrow emigrants, which explains why there can be accessory spleens within the peritoneal ligaments associated with the spleen.

   e. False The cortex develops from the mesoderm, and the medulla from the neural crest. The fetal suprarenal gland is a relatively large abdominal organ prior to birth, after which it regresses to reach adult proportions.

3. The gonads:
  a. Form as part of the primitive kidney system initially.
  b. Acquire their germ cells from the yolk sac.
  c. Develop in conjunction with a duct system which is part of the intermediate mesoderm.
  d. Migrate to their adult position following the mesonephric ridge.
  e. In the male descend through the inguinal canal before birth.

3. a. False Although the development of the two is
spatiotemporally related, the two systems are
separate. The kidney starts as a pronephros high on
the future abdominal wall, and progresses caudally,
becoming the mesonephros, and finally evolves in
the pelvis as the metanephros. The kidney is
derived from intermediate mesoderm. The gonad
arises from migrating primordial germ cells from
the endoderm of the yolk sac and the gut, into
tissues from the coelomic epithelium, thus forming
the genital ridges. Gonad development is associated
with duct development. The duct of the
mesonephros becomes associated with the
developing gonad in the male, whereas in the
female a new duct appears from the coelomic
epithelium, the paramesonephric duct.

b. True The germ cells begin to appear in the genital ridges
at about the sixth week of development.

c. False The duct systems are different in the two sexes.
In the male, the duct of the mesonephros, from the
intermediate mesoderm, becomes the duct of the
gonad, the ductus deferens. In the female, the
paramesonephric duct arises as a separate duct
from the coelomic epithelium. The mesonephric
duct in the female largely regresses, with only
epoöphoron and paroöphoron persisting between
the two layers of the broad ligament. In the male,
a small portion of the paramesonephric duct
remains as the prostatic utricle.

d. False Migration of the gonads to their adult position
follows the gubernaculum, a band of mesenchyme
passing from the caudal tip of the developing
gonad to the labia in the female or scrotum in the
male. In both sexes, therefore, the migration of the
gubernaculum passes through the inguinal canal.
However, in the female, the descent of the ovary is
arrested in the pelvis.

e. True The testes pass into the scrotum during the last
month of gestation.

4. With regard to the pharyngeal or branchial arches:
  a. The cartilage of the first arch is called Reichert's cartilage.
  b. The mesoderm of the second arch gives rise to muscle supplied by the maxillary division of the third cranial nerve.
  c. The palatine tonsils are derived from the endoderm of the second pharyngeal pouch.
  d. A branchial cyst forms from the persistence of the epicardial ridge.
  e. The only blood vessel remaining from the fifth aortic arch on the right side is the proximal part of the subclavian artery.

5. With regard to the respiratory system:
  a. The lung primordia grow into the pleuroperitoneal canals.
  b. The lungs are not fully mature until approximately 7 years of age.
  c. The lung buds arise from the mesodermal germ layer.
  d. Fluid in the lungs at the time of birth is reabsorbed by the pleural membranes.
  e. The pulmonary arteries develop *in situ* between the heart and the lungs.

4. a. False The first arch cartilage is called Meckel's cartilage. Reichert's cartilage is in the second arch. In both cases the cartilage disappears, forming ligaments – the sphenomandibular and stylohyoid ligaments, respectively.

    b. False The muscle of the second (hyoid) arch is supplied by the facial nerve. The maxillary division of the trigeminal nerve (the fifth cranial nerve) supplies skin over the face. There is no maxillary division of the third (oculomotor nerve).

    c. True The palatine tonsils are derived from the second pharyngeal arch. The epithelial lining of the developing pharynx proliferates to form buds within the mesenchyme, and into which mesodermal tissue grows to form the tonsillar tissue.

    d. False Branchial cysts arise as a result of the failure of the second arch to overgrow the third and fourth arches. A narrow canal thus persists which can open on to the surface of the neck just anterior to the sternocleidomastoid muscle.

    e. False The fifth aortic arches never really develop. The right proximal side of the subclavian artery arises from the fourth right aortic arch.

5. a. False The lung primordia grow into the pericardioperitoneal canals, part of the intraembryonic coelom.

    b. True Further bifurcation of the respiratory tree to form more alveolar sacs continues into early childhood.

    c. False The lung buds arise from the endoderm of the foregut, though they grow into surrounding mesenchyme tissue derived from the lateral plate.

    d. False Fluid from the lungs is either swallowed or absorbed by the capillary bed, or by the numerous lymphatics. Of course, much fluid is expelled from the lungs as the infant is compressed during its passage through the birth canal.

    e. False These vessels arise from the sixth aortic arches.

6. **With regard to the fibrosis of various structures, ducts and vessels in the fetus:**
   a. The right umbilical vein becomes the ligamentum arteriosum.
   b. The allantois becomes the medial umbilical ligament.
   c. The stylohyoid ligament was initially derived from Reichert's cartilage.
   d. Part of the paramesonephric duct persists in the adult as the epoöphoron and the paroöphoron in the broad ligament.
   e. The vitellointestinal duct persists as the vermiform appendix.

6. a. False The right umbilical vein disappears, whereas the
left carries oxygenated blood from the placenta to
the liver, and after birth fibroses to become the
ligamentum teres. The ligamentum arteriosum is the
fibrosed remnant of the ductus arteriosus.
   b. False The allantois becomes the *median* umbilical
ligament. The medial umbilical ligaments are the
fibrosed remnants of the right and left umbilical
arteries.
   c. True The cartilage of this arch also gives rise to the
stapes, the styloid process of the temporal bone,
and the lesser horn and upper part of the hyoid
bone.
   d. False The paramesonephric duct becomes the uterus and
upper vagina. It is part of the persisting
mesonephric duct which becomes the epoöphoron
and paroöphoron.
   e. False The vitellointestinal (vitelline) duct may persist as
Meckel's diverticulum. The appendix is derived
from the tip of the developing caecum. The
connection between the two is that the pain of an
inflamed Meckel's diverticulum and that of acute
appendicitis in its early stages are both referred to
the umbilical region of the abdominal wall.

7. **With regard to congenital anomalies:**
   a. Fallot's tetralogy is characterized by an overriding aorta, hypertrophy of the left ventricle, an atrial septal defect and pulmonary infundibular stenosis.
   b. An omphalocoele is where the intestinal loops fail to enter into the physiological hernia.
   c. Oligohydramnios results from bilateral renal agenesis.
   d. Horseshoe kidney is found in about 1 in 600 people.
   e. A cleft palate is of genetic aetiology.

7. a. False Fallot's tetralogy is characterized by an overriding
aorta and hypertrophy of the *right* ventricle,
because of increase in pressure in this chamber.
This is caused by the interventricular septal defect.
Pulmonary infundibular stenosis is also present.

b. False An omphalocoele is where the intestinal loops
herniated from the midgut fail to return, and
remain as an amnion-covered sac in the
extraembryonic coelom in the umbilical cord, lying
on the ventral abdominal wall.

c. True Bilateral renal agenesis leads to oligohydramnios
because the fetus 'drinks' amniotic fluid, but cannot
excrete it, thus the volume of fluid in the amniotic
cavity is small.

d. True This anomaly results from fusion of the lower poles
of the developing metanephros as it rises from its
original pelvic position. As a consequence of the
presence of kidney tissue in the midline, there may
be pressure on the inferior vena cava, with resulting
oedema of the lower limbs. Patients with a
horseshoe kidney can also present with recurrent
urinary tract infections, pain in the loins and a
tender abdomen. The condition is usually detected
in childhood, but may be asymptomatic.

e. True Affecting nearly 1 in 1000 live births, and more
common in males than females, it is often
accompanied by a cleft lip (hare lip). Failure of
fusion of the palatine shelves, or of the primary
and secondary palates, is the cause. Environmental
factors may also play a role.

8. In developing limbs:
    a. The apex of the limb is known as the apical ectodermal plateau.
    b. Amelia is the congenital absence of a limb.
    c. Syndactyly is the presence of extra fingers or toes.
    d. Polydactyly is where there is an extra toe or finger and the additional digit acquires anomalous muscular attachments.
    e. Meromelia is where the hand or foot is attached to the trunk via an irregularly shaped, usually quite short, bone.

9. With regard to the formation of the placenta:
    a. Tertiary chorionic villi differ from secondary chorionic villi merely by the presence of blood vessels.
    b. Primary chorionic villi contain only syncytiotrophoblast.
    c. The intervillous space contains fetal blood.
    d. The decidua basalis and the chorion laeve constitute the placenta.
    e. The umbilical cord contains a loose connective tissue called Merton's jelly.

8. a. False The apex of the limb is known as the apical ectodermal *ridge*.

b. True The term is derived from the Greek word *melos* which means limb, and has been associated in the past with use of the drug thalidomide during early pregnancy.

c. False Syndactyly is the presence of webs of skin between the fingers or toes to give a webbed hand or foot appearance. Polydactyly is the presence of additional digits.

d. False Polydactylous digits do not normally carry muscular attachments.

e. True Sometimes the whole of the limb is present but in miniature form; this is micromelia.

9. a. True Tertiary and secondary chorionic villi both contain an outer covering of syncytiotrophoblast and an inner layer of cytotrophoblast. In the tertiary villi, however, angiogenesis occurs.

b. False Primary chorionic villi contain an outer layer of syncytiotrophoblast, and an inner core of cytotrophoblast. The latter constitutes the main bulk of the villi.

c. False The intervillous space contains maternal blood. There is always a little intermixing, however. Indeed, it is possible to find maternal and fetal blood cells circulating in the fetal and maternal circulation respectively.

d. False It is the decidua basalis and the chorion *frondosum* which constitute the placenta.

e. False The umbilical cord contains a loose connective tissue called Wharton's jelly. This was discovered by Thomas Wharton, of St Thomas's Hospital, London, in 1656. His name is also associated with the submandibular duct.

10. **The developing coelomic cavity:**
    a. Is lined by extraembryonic mesoderm.
    b. Is divided by the pericardioperitoneal folds.
    c. Is divided by the septum transversum which is derived from somatopleuric mesoderm.
    d. Is divided by the diaphragm which is in part made up of the mesoduodenum.
    e. Is divided by the diaphragm which is in part made up of the occipital myotomes.

10. a. False It is lined by *intraembryonic mesoderm*, the somatopleuric lateral plate mesoderm. The splanchnopleuric mesoderm invests the viscera.
   b. False It is divided by the pleuropericardial folds between the pericardial and pleural cavities, and by the pleuroperitoneal folds between the pleural and peritoneal cavities. Lying between the two are the pericardioperitoneal canals, the future pleural cavities.
   c. False It is divided by the septum transversum but this is derived from unsegmented mesoderm which initially lies cranial to the prochordal plate.
   d. False It is divided by the diaphragm but it is the meso-oesophagus which partly forms the structure.
   e. False It is divided by the diaphragm but the latter is invaded by myotomes from the third, fourth and fifth cervical regions, hence its motor innervation by the phrenic nerve and the curious pattern of referred pain associated with afflictions of the diaphragm.